Dear Mary:

May we continue together
to stay
on the ethical way!

12/11/01

The Ethical Way

The Jossey-Bass Managed Behavioral Healthcare Library

Michael A. Freeman, General Editor

Marketing for Therapists:
A Handbook for Success in Managed Care

Jeri Davis, Editor

The Computerization of Behavioral Healthcare:
How to Enhance Clinical Practice, Management,
and Communications

Tom Trabin, Editor

Behavioral Risk Management: How to Avoid Preventable
Losses from Mental Health Problems in the Workplace

Rudy M. Yandrick

Training Behavioral Healthcare Professionals:
Higher Learning in the Era of Managed Care

James M. Schuster, Mark R. Lovell,
and Anthony M. Trachta, Editors

The Ethical Way: Challenges and Solutions for
Managed Behavioral Healthcare

H. Steven Moffic

The Complete Capitation Handbook

Gayle L. Zieman, Editor

Inside Outcomes: The National Review of
Behavioral Healthcare Outcomes

Tom Trabin, Michael A. Freeman, and Michael Pallak

Managed Behavioral Healthcare: History, Models,
Strategic Challenges, and Future Course

Michael A. Freeman and Tom Trabin

Behavioral Group Practice Performance Characteristics:
The Council of Group Practices Benchmarking Study

Allen Daniels, Teresa Kramer, and Nalini Mahesh

How to Respond to Managed Behavioral Healthcare:
A Workbook Guide for Your Organization

Barbara Mauer, Dale Jarvis, Richard Mockler, and Tom Trabin

H. Steven Moffic

Foreword by Michael A. Freeman,
General Editor

The Ethical Way

Challenges and Solutions for
Managed Behavioral Healthcare

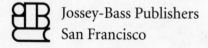 Jossey-Bass Publishers
San Francisco

Substantial discounts on bulk quantities of Jossey-Bass books are available to corporations, professional associations, and other organizations. For details and discount information, contact the special sales department at Jossey-Bass Inc., Publishers (415) 433–1740; Fax (800) 605–2665.

For sales outside the United States, please contact your local Simon & Schuster International Office.

Jossey-Bass Web address: http://www.josseybass.com

 Manufactured in the United States of America on Lyons Falls Turin Book. This paper is acid-free and 100 percent totally chlorine-free.

Library of Congress Cataloging-in-Publication Data

Moffic, H. Steven.
    The ethical way : challenges and solutions for managed behavioral healthcare / H. Steven Moffic.
        p.   cm. — (The Jossey-Bass managed behavioral healthcare library)
    Includes bibliographical references and index.
    ISBN 0-7879-0841-X
    1. Managed mental health care—Moral and ethical aspects.
  I. Title. II. Series.
  RC455.2.E8M64   1997
  174'.2—dc21   96-53565

FIRST EDITION
HB Printing 10 9 8 7 6 5 4 3 2 1

Contents

To Rusti

Bringing sunshine every day is The Ethical Way

—∿— Foreword

Behavioral healthcare has changed. The old and once familiar professional landscape now seems altered and disorienting. The familiar landmarks that were well known to mental health administrators, clinicians, insurance executives, employee assistance program directors, and academic researchers are fading off the map. Vanishing or gone are the employers who did not pay attention to healthcare costs, the insurance plans that would reimburse on a fee-for-service basis, the hospitals with beds filled with patients whose coverage encouraged long lengths of stay, the solo clinicians with full practices of affluent patients seeking long-term insight-oriented therapy, and the community mental health centers that worked in a system of their own.

The scenery of today is different. Health maintenance organizations and managed behavioral health plans have replaced the insurance companies. Employers and purchasing cooperatives are bypassing even these new organizations and purchasing directly from providers. Clinicians are forming group practices. Groups are affiliating with facilities. Facilities are forming integrated delivery systems. Integrated delivery systems are building organized systems of care that include insurance, care management, and service delivery functions. Information systems are linking payers, managers, and providers into coordinated and comprehensive systems with new levels of accountability. The boundaries of the public sector are eroding, and the distinction between public and private has become more difficult to perceive.

Adjusting to this "brave new world" is challenging, and many mental health professionals are being tempted to give up and opt out now. But for most of us, the challenge is worth facing. While this period is fraught with difficulty and risk, there are also a number of opportunities. Whenever a paradigm shifts, those having a stake in the previous paradigm risk losing their place in the one that emerges. The Jossey-Bass Managed Behavioral Healthcare Library will help you identify and confront the challenges you will face as the prevailing healthcare paradigms change. Moreover, the volumes in this library will provide you with pragmatic strategies and solutions that you can call upon to sustain your importance in the healthcare systems of the future.

In spite of the upheavals transforming the behavioral healthcare enterprise in this country, many of its basic goals remain the same. In fact, managed behavioral healthcare has come about largely because our previous way of doing things failed to solve fundamental problems related to the cost, quality, accessibility, and outcomes of care. "Managed behavioral healthcare"—whatever this concept may eventually come to mean—holds out the promise of affordable, appropriate, and effective mental health and addiction treatment services for all. The various initiatives and efforts that are under way to reach this new service plateau will result in a vast array of professional opportunities for the behavioral healthcare specialists whose talents are required to make this promise come true.

By reading the books and reports in the Managed Behavioral Healthcare Library, you will learn how to respond to the perils and possibilities presented by today's shift to managed behavioral healthcare. The authors of this book and of the other volumes in this series recognize the need for direct and pragmatic solutions to the challenges posed by the changing paradigms of behavioral healthcare financing and services. To help you meet this need and obtain the resources and solutions you require, each chapter of each publication is written by an outstanding expert who can communicate in a pragmatic style to help you make a difference and meet each of the key challenges posed by the new landscape in behavioral healthcare.

This volume and the others planned for the series help you improve your effectiveness at pricing, financing, and delivering high-quality, cost-effective care. Future volumes will also provide straight-forward solutions to the ethical challenges of managed behavioral healthcare and offer advice about practice management and marketing during a period of industry consolidation. You can look forward to still other books and reports about developing and managing a group practice, creating workplace-based behavioral healthcare programs, measuring outcomes, computerizing delivery systems, and ways of "benchmarking" in order to compare your organization or practice with others that face similar challenges.

Because the landscape of behavioral healthcare is in flux, professionals in the field need to be aware of alternative scenarios of the future and develop the skill sets for success within each one. For behavioral healthcare leaders, it is critical to have the vision to select the best options that accord with shared values and to have the skills to put these possibilities into practice. For this reason, the themes of vision, action, and results are incorporated into the volumes you read in the Managed Behavioral Healthcare Library.

VISION

In the context of the current debate and upheavals in healthcare, we have seen broad agreement regarding the importance of behavioral health scrutiny at an affordable price for all Americans. The Managed Behavioral Healthcare Library offers publications that show how universal coverage for affordable, appropriate, accessible, and effective mental health and addiction treatment benefits and services can be achieved.

METHODS

How can we put into operation the new paradigms, the new models and systems of care needed to make the promise of managed care come true? New methods of benefit administration and health services delivery will be required to implement this vision within realistic financial limits.

At the broadest level, these methods include the core technologies used to manage benefits, care, and the health status of individuals and defined populations. At the level of frontline operations, these methods include continuous quality improvement, process reengineering, outcomes management, public-private integration, computerization, and delivery system reconfiguration in the context of capitation financing. These are the areas in which the Managed Behavioral Healthcare Library helps you build skill sets.

New methods of direct clinical care are also required. Instead of treating episodes of illness, clinicians in future managed and integrated behavioral healthcare systems will use disease-state management methods to reduce morbidity and mortality for individuals and for groups. The Managed Behavioral Healthcare Library provides frontline clinicians and delivery system managers with the skills that will enable our healthcare systems to truly provide scientifically validated bio-psycho-social treatment of choice in behavioral healthcare.

ACTION AND RESULTS

Knowing that we are in a period of change, and even having the desire to make the changes that are needed, makes little difference without actions based on methods that can produce results. Because you take action and produce results through day-in, day-out application of your professional expertise, the Managed Behavioral Healthcare Library is action oriented, to provide the greatest possible benefit to you and your colleagues.

—⁓—

Restructuring of the behavioral healthcare enterprise cannot take place without raising profound ethical challenges. How does a clinician balance the patient's right to confidentiality with society's need for outcome data to determine treatments of choice? What should a provider do when benefits expire yet patients still require treatment? How does one respond to financial incentives to provide too little care, or too much?

Though these challenges may be profound, they are also immediate and require pragmatic solutions that can be applied in the day in, day out delivery of mental health services. This volume, *The Ethical Way,* is perhaps the first to confront the most critical and commonly experienced of these challenges head on and provide pragmatic solutions in the process.

Structured as an "easy read" novel that walks one through the process of creating an imaginary managed behavioral healthcare company, *The Ethical Way* leads professionals through basic ethical principles, issues related to gatekeeping and informed consent, the challenges of confidentiality and financial influence, and ethical dilemmas encountered while delivering care. It also addresses the ethics of utilization review and anticipates future challenges.

Throughout this journey, a broad and diverse panel of industry experts has joined the story to comment on most chapters, yielding the insight and wisdom of consumer advocates, managed care executives, providers, government officials, medical ethicists, and legal scholars. Taken together, the author and the discussants have created one of the most useful, accessible, and results-oriented portraits of managed behavioral healthcare ethics that is currently available.

As a volume in the Managed Behavioral Healthcare Library, this book is certain to make a significant contribution to the field, and to the daily practice of those who read it. Under the cost-containment pressures of our current environment, the need for a solid and understandable architecture of ethics and values is imperative, and this exegesis goes a long way toward meeting this objective.

We have designed this book, along with the other volumes in the Managed Behavioral Healthcare Library, to provide the information and inspiration essential for all professionals who want to understand the challenges and opportunities available today.

Tiburon, California   MICHAEL A. FREEMAN, M.D.
February 1997

⸺ Preface

When I was asked to consider writing this book, I confirmed my strong sense that there was no other book available on this topic. Yes, there were scattered articles on various ethical issues in managed behavioral healthcare, but no comprehensive publication. How puzzling that seemed! After all, for the last decade or so, we have been living through the greatest changes in health and behavioral healthcare systems that have ever taken place in so short a period of time. And the transition has certainly not been smooth. In reactions from those pro and con managed care, ethical issues have always been in the forefront, ranging from concern over the business aspects of managed care to the effects on patient care, with clinicians often feeling caught in the middle. So one would have thought there would have been several books on ethical issues in managed behavioral healthcare by now.

As I got to work, the reason for this omission became more readily apparent. The ethical issues are immense, complex, and daunting. Taking sides would be easy but not fair or conducive to presenting a balanced and comprehensive consideration. Potential readership could include business leaders, governmental healthcare administrators, administrators of managed care companies, mental health clinicians of all disciplines, students, ethicists, and politicians, so a simple approach geared to one perspective would not suffice.

I felt I could be fair, as I had been involved in mental health ethical deliberations for a long time and worked in an academic setting that had been interested in a scholarly approach to managed behavioral healthcare. But even with my background, how could I develop such a book to give the subject its due? Eventually, several organizing principles emerged.

First, I needed to give a sense of my own ethical struggles on the topic to enable the reader to understand some of my perspective. Self-disclosure could also counter the tendency toward secrecy in many managed care organizations.

Then, to go beyond general ethical analysis, it seemed useful to try to make the everyday ethical struggles that we all have come alive. To do that, I decided to tell the fictional story of an emerging managed behavioral healthcare company, supplemented by—and interwoven with—ethical analyses of the issues. The company is a small one, designed to highlight challenges that will emerge in any managed care system. It has a business leader and a healthcare leader, to reflect both business and behavioral healthcare ethics.

Our imaginary company grapples with the range of ethical challenges, from the way a company approaches ethical issues to the specific ethical problems it encounters in individual patient care interactions. Along the way, each major challenge is put into a historical perspective for context and to see what's new. We end with ethical hopes and solutions for the future.

The overriding principle was to present all of this with an idealistic tinge. The story is not one that is supposed to reflect reality precisely. Rather, it is humbly designed to show how our ethical challenges might be solved in an ethical way.

It is also not the only story that could be told or the only ethical way that can be taken. Consequently, brief commentaries by experts from a variety of backgrounds have been added throughout.

So, come meet Evelyn, Adam, Buddy, The Bear, Peter, Sun-Yu, and the rest in The Ethical Way as we begin our journey.

ACKNOWLEDGMENTS

Where does one ethically start acknowledgments in writing a book like this? With one's parents? A demanding high school writing teacher like Elaine Grauer? A creative writing class at Michigan? Unobtainable models on ethics like Hippocrates? The publish-or-perish expectations of academic psychiatry? Patients, colleagues, and managed care innovators who challenged ethical assumptions?

I'm not sure, so I'll just continue from the beginning of this project. Thanks to James Sabin for sending me on this ethical way in more ways than one, and for believing I could find my own way. Much gratitude to Alan Rinzler, my editor at Jossey-Bass, who could take my dim subconscious ideas and almost stream-of-consciousness writing, then shape that into whatever worth they had. Appreciation also goes to Michael Freeman, who serves as general editor for the Managed Behavioral Healthcare Library series, not only for his helpful suggestions, but especially for his leadership of the Institute of Behavioral Healthcare, which has filled crucial niches in education on managed behavioral healthcare neglected by more traditional institutions.

Finally, much help was provided in my everyday life to support this endeavor. Many typists worked patiently with the changes along the way: Sally Krochalk, Krystal Wiedower, and Mary Kusz especially. The department of psychiatry administration at the Medical College of Wisconsin provided all the help they could. Ross Carter and Charlene Carter gave invaluable feedback at a crucial stage in the process. In addition, a lifelong closest friend, Barry Marcus, was struggling with the challenges of his institution undergoing a managed care transformation while I was working on the book, and this provided a special, poignant urgency to look for the ethical way. Personal ethics begins at home in one's family of origin, but in my case it is enhanced by the standards Evan, Stacia, Rusti, and I try to meet in the Moffic, a.k.a. Rustevie, family.

Milwaukee, Wisconsin
February 1997

H. STEVEN MOFFIC

The Ethical Way

Introduction

I must confess.

It was in 1989 when I first encountered my own ethical and legal challenges in managed behavioral healthcare. I remember all too clearly the first time I had some administrative responsibility for a managed care system in addition to my usual clinical responsibilities to patients. That was about seven years ago. I had come to Milwaukee to work as a tenured professor and director of development for the Department of Psychiatry at the Medical College of Wisconsin. A major thrust of the development was designed to be managed care. Some of the rest of my time was to go into some "private practice" type of clinical work.

I had come from the public psychiatric sector. From academic community mental health, in fact, although that terminology is rapidly becoming obsolete. That work had been at Baylor College of Medicine in Houston, where a major part of my job had been as clinical director for a community mental health center covering a catchment area of about 500,000 people. I was used to providing what was possible under very limiting financial circumstances, a challenge I actually looked forward to. Rationing, fair or not, has always been a

factor in the public sector. I felt some kind of a moral imperative to do the best possible for those who were usually neglected: the poor, the chronics, the minorities.

Some of the reasons to do so probably have to do with personal psychodynamics. Some of it must also have to do with my Jewish ethnic background, which emphasizes *tikkun olam,* to heal and transform the world. Some of it likely comes from valued role models during my undergraduate and graduate years.

So, in some regards, managed care did not appear to me to be so different from the public sector. As if the public sector had come to the middle class, if you will. Maybe that's what all the uproar was about, that the middle class and their clinicians were faced with the kind of treatment limits previously reserved for the poor. In managed care, similar limits would exist on how much and what kind of treatment would be permitted. So why not try it and see what it was like? Maybe something could be learned in managed care that would eventually be helpful in the public sector.

One of my colleagues in the public sector had been advocating that we should somehow expand into health maintenance organizations, in that managed care was the biggest thing coming. However, when he was indicted for embezzling funds from the county, I wondered if his interest in managed care might have been due to the potential for big financial gain, one way or another.

In any case, taking this new job caused some concern from others for my career, since managed care wasn't exactly popular in academic medicine. But I did have the support of a courageous and visionary chairman at work and a loving and intuitive wife at home, so I jumped in feet first, or as some would say, backside first. On my first day in the new work setting, I was offered the possibility of developing and administrating a full at-risk subcapitated managed care system for the complete mental health treatment of about 10,000 people (or *covered lives,* to use the terminology). The capitation rate was about $3.50 per member per month. So we had over $400,000 a year to take care of all the mental healthcare needs of 10,000 working-class people. This shouldn't be too hard, I thought, though any catastrophic cases could pose a big financial risk. But even with family members included, this should be a relatively healthy population compared to what I was used to. So we took the contract, even with no system in place, just a strategy of somehow adapting community mental health principles to a different kind of population. Anxiety was replaced with excitement. So far, so good.

However, my first inkling that this new managed care endeavor would bring unusual challenges was when the other administrators and I were discussing financial projections for this first contract. Since there could be leftover money from this capitation, I was offered the possibility of receiving a percentage of any profits.

At first, I wasn't even sure what that meant. Profits in mental health? In the public sector, we always struggled just to make ends meet, bringing in our own old household supplies if necessary. And weren't profits supposed to occur only in businesses? Salaries in medicine? Sure. Fee-for-service in medicine? Sure, at least if the fees were reasonable. Hospital profits? Maybe that made sense, if the hospital wasn't called a "not-for-profit" hospital. But profits in an academic institution trying to serve society by providing the best education, newest research ideas, and most advanced treatment techniques?

Then someone said, "Well, it's really savings we're talking about, not profits. And lots of managed care companies do this." Savings in the sense of watching how much was being spent. Was that what he meant? And how did that apply to what we were going to do? I would soon enough find out. Although tempted and appreciative of the offer, for the meantime I decided to turn down the "percentage of profit" possibility. I had a reasonable salary and enough to worry about already. And I silently wondered, with some relief, why I wasn't also asked to take a risk of salary reduction if we lost money.

MANAGED CARE FROM AN IVORY TOWER

My goal, I thought at the time, was to study managed care from the ivory tower—from the neutral perspective of an academic institution. What was really good about managed care, and what was really bad?

On one hand, there were local and national managed care companies changing the face of health delivery and seeing their stock prices rise on Wall Street. If they weren't doing any real research to see how they were doing as far as clinical outcomes, so what? The payers were starting to save money, at a time when our nation's healthcare costs were escalating. And if fees were being cut to providers, wasn't it about time? How could some of those surgeons charge so much for a procedure, even if it was lifesaving? And how could hospitals slip in $100 charges for two aspirin? And surely peer review had turned into a good-old-boy, pat-you-on-the-back maneuver. How come it took so long to catch any of those clinicians who engaged in sexual relations with patients? Was interminable psychoanalysis really medically necessary?

On the other hand, you had your academic medical and graduate mental health institutions of psychiatry, psychology, social work, and nursing. So far, they had washed their hands of managed care. Maybe not up-to-date, but at least they were free of any contamination from the managed care craze that was sweeping the country. They didn't even seem interested in researching the outcomes of managed care systems versus traditional fee-for-service care. They hoped managed care was a fad that would soon die. After all, hadn't all previous attempts at healthcare reform in this country died?

Opinions, moreover, varied greatly. In a national survey of academic chairs of departments of psychiatry we were soon to do, we received such comments about managed care as:

"We have done a very poor job of developing standards of care and holding ourselves to them and managed care seems to be imposing some discipline on the system."

"Little short of disaster."

"Managed care is a concept that was born with community mental health and refined by the for-profit sector."

"Generally second-rate treatment."

"It will take some serious lawsuits to cut it down to size."

"We need another decade of experiences to make a definitive statement."

So I thought that embarking on this subcapitated managed mental healthcare contract in an academic setting was the best of both worlds. We wouldn't be overly driven by the profit motive, and we could study this managed care phenomenon in a neutral, scholarly way.

First, I even thought of a clever new name for our new system. To soften the business association of "managed" care, and to suggest an ethical concern, we decided on Humanage ("We Manage To Care"), with the accent on the first or second syllable. I thought this name was a nice contrast to the name of another local managed care company called Take Control. Our written mission statement was "The secret of managed care is in managing to care while managing the care." We even provided a patient information packet describing the benefits, our network, and the grievance procedure.

Soon I found out that this brave new managed care world wasn't exactly what I thought it was. Research was the first to go. How could we reserve and use funds for research if we weren't sure at first that we wouldn't lose money? Let's set up a reserve fund first, just in case, came the order from central administration. Education was next. Why should

our students be educated in managed care? We're interested in teaching them the best treatment, the ideal treatment, not what is only "medically necessary." Anyway, we don't teach students about systems; we teach them about psychotherapy and medication. That could be done anywhere.

I said OK. I thought later on we could easily add on the research and educational components. We did, though, include administrative costs. We settled on 15 percent, given the paperwork and utilization reviewing and network forming and credentialing we thought we had to do (at least that's what one recent continuing medical education course on managed care systems taught me). I understood that 15 percent for administration was still below the 20 to 25 percent that was mentioned for many managed care companies. Our first staff hire was someone who had a combined social work and business background and who would do both administrative and clinical work.

My Perspective as an Administrator

So we started, and I was soon to find out that not only was this brave new managed care world not what I thought it was, but that I wasn't who I thought I was. I thought that with all my psychological self-analysis and therapy, I knew pretty much who I was, at least in a professional sense. But new insights and revelations arrived quickly.

Within the first week of the contract, and without a real network of clinicians in place, a thirty-five-year-old male ended up in the hospital. As I now knew you were supposed to do in managed care, I called the attending psychiatrist to do a utilization review. I said we needed to know about the patient and the psychiatrist's treatment expectations before we could authorize payment, a payment I quickly told him would be 30 percent below his (and my) customary fee-for-service rates. I guess he had some familiarity with managed care rates, for with a quick sigh, he agreed. The hospital, also, had readily agreed to a steeply discounted rate, although I wondered why it was so easy to negotiate these rates. Should the rates have been lower all along, or was this just using excess capacity? In any case, everything seemed fine financially with this first case. We were looking at paying about $500 a day for everything. Pretty reasonable, I thought.

Then we got into what we were all about anyway, that is what was wrong with the patient and what the treatment plans were going to be. I thought this would be a little like live peer review over the phone, so it had a ring of familiarity.

The psychiatrist said it looked like a psychotic depression, with command hallucinations saying the person was greedy and bad and to kill himself. Some outpatient psychotherapy by a social worker had been started, but the patient had worsened. Seemed like a reasonable need for hospitalization to me. Then I asked what sort of treatment plan the psychiatrist had in mind and how long he expected the patient to be in the hospital. He said they probably needed a few days of observation and evaluation, that, hopefully, a one-on-one suicide watch wouldn't be needed, then to start either an antidepressant or antipsychotic medication, then start the other after a few more days, then if all went well, the patient should be ready to consider discharge in perhaps three or four weeks. A long sentence, but not bad, I thought—at least he wasn't asking for one of those canned twenty-eight-day programs that seemed to be so common for any substance abuse program. I had always been taught that observation for a few days is clinically important, perhaps in this case to rule out schizophrenia, a borderline personality disorder, substance abuse, or thyroid disease. A long shot might be a posttraumatic stress disorder. So what if the psychiatrist was a little indecisive about what kind of medication to start, though I thought the antipsychotic should be used first and perhaps quickly, and after that, a loading dose of the antidepressant nortriptyline to speed things up.

Then, in the midst of these clinical discussions and associations, an intrusive thought popped up in my mind. "Don't you know how much this is all going to cost?" a strange voice seemed to be saying to me. "He's saying maybe thirty days, and even at only $500 a day, that would be, what, $15,000?" With some quick brain computing, I realized that was almost half of our projected monthly capitated revenue—and if any one-on-ones were needed for suicide monitoring, the costs would escalate.

"One more hospitalization like this and we're already in the red," I could hear the department administrator reminding me. The administrator might even start giving his clinical advice, like "Isn't there another way to treat this depression?" Not a bad question, actually.

And what about all the outpatients, let alone day treatment? You figure, out of ten thousand people, probably around 5 percent will want or need outpatient treatment, or about five hundred. I had just heard of one whom the therapist wanted to continue in two-times-a-week psychotherapy, to continue the three-year process of dealing with anxiety to big life changes. This therapist was a psychiatrist, so we're talking about $100 an hour at discounted rates. At the requested frequency, that's $800 a month, or $10,000 a year.

My gosh, with just thirteen month-long hospitalizations and twenty two-times-a-week psychotherapy patients, there goes the whole capitation revenue. How could I even think about doing the preventive programs promised by the original health maintenance organizations, or doing the outreach to all those needing mental healthcare but reluctant to come in? Such endeavors would cost staff time, and staff time was money, of which we had a limited supply. Finally, in my financial reveries, I heard the loud, firm voice of the attending psychiatrist, "So am I authorized or not?" I felt guilty, so I quickly said OK, "but we'll call you every other day to see how the patient is doing."

Two more weeks passed. Our social worker first-line utilization reviewer felt discharge was indicated for that hospitalized patient, but the attending psychiatrist did not, so there was an appeal to me. The psychiatrist said the auditory hallucinations were virtually gone, the medication was being tolerated well, the patient seemed to have more insight, and he was beginning to be less depressed.

"So then why not discharge?" I asked.

The attending psychiatrist quickly parried with, "Well, we all know that what seems like a beginning improvement in a depressed patient can be a mask for a firm resolution to kill oneself, and now having the energy to actually do so."

"But is there any explanation you have for why that would be the case now?" I replied haughtily.

"Well, no, but maybe he wouldn't tell me, or maybe he's still hearing voices and listening to them saying to fool the psychiatrist and not tell him." It started to feel to me that we were getting nowhere, in a sparring of clinical wits, yet he had a point, so I suggested that the patient come straight from the hospital to our network clinic or start day treatment. The psychiatrist balked, feeling the patient was still at risk. Was he clinically right, clinically ignorant, too cautious, or even—I was reluctant to think—greedy?

"Well, it's up to you of course," I said, "All we're doing is authorizing payment, but it's still your medical—" (and legal, I thought) "—responsibility of whether to discharge or not. We'll also have to let the patient know."

"Let the patient know?" he exasperatingly questioned. "That's unethical. He's my patient and you can't intrude like that. You're really disrupting the patient-clinician alliance."

"Well, he does have a right to know what his insurance will pay for," I countered. I thought we could have a three-part alliance, though I realized that could complicate things by producing splitting or acting out.

"What if this was your patient? What would you do? Better yet, what if it was one of your family members insured by your system?"

That question caught me a little short emotionally. Most people want the best possible for their family.

Eventually, we both ran out of threats, agreeing on two more days and for the attending psychiatrist to follow up with the patient.

Our system then settled into some kind of routine, simultaneously trying to triage patients, monitor their care, and keep track of our expenses. Many times, the treatment we monitored seemed appropriate. Brief therapy for circumscribed problems. The right doses of antidepressants for major depression. However, at times we were also horrified. Drug cocktails, with inadequate doses of any medication, for unclear diagnoses. Hypnotherapy with consequent worsening of dissociative symptoms. Allegations of seductive behavior on the part of a respected psychotherapist. Family, group, and individual psychotherapy with no improvement in symptoms of what sounded like attention deficit disorder in the identified adolescent patient. Treatment plans that gave "my experience with such problems" as the justification for treatment, rather than literature, consultation, or even patient request. Information provided that we later found out was distorted. I was a little surprised at how easy it soon became to "just say no" to authorizing payment for such questionable treatment. Yet I couldn't help wondering if I was qualified to make such judgments, or was "identifying with the aggressor"—or, in other words, was I just acting as mean and authoritarian as other controversial reviewers and managers I had heard about?

We also had some pleasant surprises. There were many clinicians we hadn't known of who worked in the community, carefully but quickly making diagnoses, taking costs into account, presenting options to patients, and achieving obvious improvement. We also found that just the presence or threat of utilization review seemed to be changing the amount of treatment being provided. Once clinicians learned about our review mechanisms, their inpatient length of stays and number of outpatient visits seemed to decrease almost magically. It did make us wonder, though, why the clinicians hadn't made those changes without being reviewed.

As time went on, we decided to start hiring a multidisciplinary treatment staff to supplement our community network clinicians.

That way, clinicians with different skills could work together with a common goal of cost-effective treatment.

My Perspective as a Provider

The horror stories, surprises, and challenges to my knowledge all combined to shake up my original clinical and ethical assumptions. No longer was I so sure how many days of hospitalization should routinely be expected for certain conditions. Why couldn't we try more loading doses of medication for depression or mania in the hospital? How brief should brief therapy be? Was it really best—or even cost-effective—for psychiatrists to triage all new patients? Could intermittent, developmentally oriented psychotherapy be more cost-effective over the long run? Had our traditional fee-for-service payment systems motivated unnecessary treatment at times?

Such questions were turned on their heads when I was the treating provider of my private patients dealing with another managed care company. Around the same time, I had a similar male patient who seemed depressed and suicidal and was carrying a gun. I thought hospitalization was needed, so the hospital admissions office called the out-of-town managed care company for approval. They asked to talk to me for clinical information. I asked to whom I was talking. A name was given, but not a discipline, citing "confidentiality." I knew about ethical guidelines for confidentiality, as privacy has traditionally been viewed as so important in psychiatry, but this use of "confidentiality" was something different. A series of questions ensued that sounded like a checklist. I started to feel more and more frustrated, as the questions seemed trivial and unimportant.

"Could you provide me your admissions criteria?" I asked. (Even though our own system did not have such criteria, I had heard other companies did.)

"Proprietary information, sorry," was the reply. So the questions continued. One caught me short: "Are there bullets in the gun?" I realized I didn't know, but wondered whether that was important. More questions about whether there was enough of a support network to watch the patient, whether there was any drug abuse, and whether there was a history of sexual abuse. This interrogation felt something like an unwanted second opinion. While the questions had some relevance, I worried about confidentiality—I wasn't sure the patient would have wanted so much personal information to go out, but at least this reviewer was from out of town. The admission was finally approved; I got one week. It proved to be enough to reduce the suicide risk and the depression, so I didn't consider appealing the one-week limit.

Then I had another outpatient who had a history of self-mutilation and repetitive abusive relationships. The patient surely needed twice-weekly therapy. I felt once a week would not give enough continuity to prevent symptom exacerbations. My treatment plan requested twice-weekly therapy for at least six months; it was approved for once a week for three months, as I really couldn't cite any studies to prove that such patients usually did better with more intensive therapy. I told the patient and discussed what I thought we could still accomplish. Though agreeable to try what was approved, the patient did cut herself before the next session. I wondered and offered an interpretation that the approval process felt abusive and a boundary violation of confidentiality. It seemed to help the patient, but we were still stuck with once-a-week therapy. What would I do, I pondered, if ongoing treatment was denied when I felt the patient wasn't ready? Could she self-pay? How much would be sufficient to me? What should be our therapeutic goals? If I protested too much, would these other managed care companies remove me as a network provider?

Now, at the same time that I was seeing patients in my own practice, some of whom were part of other managed care systems, I was also seeing patients in our own capitated multidisciplinary system. With these patients, I was starting to second-guess and limit my own treatment. Was I now realizing that I had taken too much of my own treatment decision making for granted over the years, or was I just being more cost-conscious to save our system more money? Was it unethical to be so influenced by the financial parameters of the patient's payment system when making treatment decisions?

STRUGGLING FOR NEW VALUES

I started to wonder why I was having all these questions. I was also perplexed that my attitude and reactions seemed to be greatly affected by where I was operating within the managed care system. What was happening to my values? To medicine's ethics? What were the laws?

I had taught and written about psychiatric ethical issues for years by this point, and had felt comfortable with how our profession had developed its values. The mental health field had various ethical codes, ranging from the Hippocratic Oath (which many medical schools no longer even ask their students to take) to the codes of psychiatrists, psychologists, social workers, and nurses. But there were some obvious guidelines that all clinicians seemed to remember, such as:

- The patient comes first, but keep in mind societal needs, especially with dangerous patients.
- Tell the patient as much as possible about treatment to support informed consent, even though a psychiatric condition could affect the rational processing of such information.
- Promise and keep absolute confidentiality, unless someone's life is in danger (other than, of course, writing a patient's diagnosis on an insurance form, and, if necessary, don't make it sound too bad), and don't forget the Tarasoff legal ruling, which is about the duty to warn of a patient's violent intentions.
- Do not use patients for financial gain, beyond acceptable community rates for services.
- No sexual or close relationships with patients, at least during treatment and for some time—if not forever—thereafter.

Now it started to seem like some of this ethical ground was turning into mud or quicksand. Some of those guidelines weren't so obvious anymore, and a new set of assumptions was required:

- Try to keep the patient's needs foremost, but don't forget there are only so many resources that have to be spread out for all those in need.
- Tell the patient as much as possible about treatment options, but the legal contract with the managed care company may forbid criticizing the company's policies or directives to the patient or anyone else (the so-called gag rule).
- Try to keep utmost confidentiality, but if you want to get paid by the managed care company, you'd better tell the reviewer about the patient's life, sex life included.
- Do not use the patient for personal gain, but remember that if your company saves money on a capitated contract, you might get a bonus.
- No sexual or close relationships with patients, at least during treatment and for some time—if not forever—thereafter.

At least the last guideline was the same! And maybe the close scrutiny of utilization reviewers could be reducing transgression of this guideline.

But since our medical and mental health professions had not adopted official new ethical guidelines, and no new medical laws had been passed that I knew of, what was happening?

THE SITUATION TODAY

It's now about seven years later. Managed care, in all its varieties, has continued to rapidly absorb more market share. Over 50 million people are now enrolled in HMOs and 76 million in PPOs. It seems to be getting harder and harder to define managed care—though being an organized system with some sort of management activities in place to deliver cost-effective care, still seems to fit. It appears that managed care has gone through four stages, from minimal case management to extensive managed care penetration with consolidation of systems of care for capitation. While different geographical areas of the country are in different stages, perhaps now some parts of the country are even entering a fifth stage, characterized by horizontally and vertically integrated large systems with direct contracts to businesses.

In the United States, the percentage of covered lives under managed care systems continues to escalate. Large companies merge. New managed care organizational models continue to appear, including large provider alliances. New payment mechanisms are being tried, such as paying clinicians a flat fee for outpatient treatment over a year, no matter what may turn out to be needed for treatment. Multimillion dollar executive salaries are disclosed. All that seems constant is ambivalent and extreme reactions, as managed care was described at a recent psychiatric conference as "a Jekyll and Hyde," "an avalanche," "all about Wall Street," "the best we can do," and "the Antichrist." The American Psychiatric Association's Hotline, designed to process managed care complaints, has evolved into a Helpline that also helps psychiatrists adapt to managed care. In the many organizations of the various mental health disciplines, intense political struggles between pro and con managed care constituents are commonplace. A professional and consumer national Mental Health Coalition has arisen to protest denial of psychotherapy. Sessions on ethical issues in managed care seem to draw larger and larger audiences at professional meetings.

My own managed care program is still in operation, though we have a new name. To my dismay, during an administrative change a few years ago, we came to be known as Behavioral Health Services instead of Humanage. We're now averaging a steady annual savings of about 15 percent. We pay our own psychiatrists discounted fee-for-service to see patients, with a rationale that any incentive to overtreat with fee-for-service might balance any incentive to undertreat by the capitation system. Faculty psychiatrists and psychologists provide part-time clinical care, but the bulk of the clinical care—especially outpatient—is provided by full-time employed master's-level clinicians, who receive a competitive salary based on twenty-eight hours a week of expected clinical productivity. We also use other mental health clinicians in the community for geographical reasons or special expertise, and pay them on a discounted fee-for-fee basis. Our hospital length of stays are down to an average of four days. Our average outpatient treatment lasts seven sessions. Both our Title 19 Aid for Families with Dependent Children patients and our commercial capitated patients are treated in the same one-tier system and have similar utilization. Some students are being educated at their request. Outcome studies are starting. No disasters are occurring. The rehospitalization rate is less than 8 percent over two years. Patient satisfaction surpasses their prior treatment system, even for the more seriously ill who had been in the public sector.

I've also had some other administrative experience in managed care outside the academic ivory tower. As part-time medical director for a local for-profit managed care organization, I have found that its system responds more quickly, is more interested in growth, and is more secretive about policies and financial considerations than our system. However, I wasn't really sure if its clinical outcomes were any worse than ours. As a member of the advisory board of another for-profit local managed care organization, one that emphasized local and national case management services, I found that it didn't seem to value questions or dissent about its operation, especially any questions about the quality of the quality assurance process or the accuracy of the marketing material. I was never quite sure whether the advisory board was disbanded or I was let go, but eventually I stopped receiving notices of future meetings. I don't remember that ethical issues were ever discussed at administrative meetings of either of these organizations.

My own clinical care is becoming similar, no matter what payment system the patient is under. I have come to find that much shorter hospitalizations, briefer medication visits, and even intermittent psychotherapy can often achieve satisfactory results for the patients and for me. My own income has increased while that of many psychiatrists has been decreasing. I enjoy that more than I think I should, but justify it by rationalizing that I was underpaid when working in community mental health all those years. I have struggled with the question of investing in for-profit managed care companies, which seem likely to do well on Wall Street, but which are reputed to prosper at the expense of patient care. After some costly delay, I decided on a health care mutual fund, which at least would invest in a whole variety of managed care companies. And I am feeling as much like a CEO as a psychiatrist.

Maybe that feeling is the answer to what was happening with our ethical issues in managed behavioral healthcare. I notice that the psychiatrist who was the head of that venerable psychiatric hospital, Sheppard Pratt in Baltimore, is now called president, medical director, and chief executive officer. Professionals are being called providers; patients are being called consumers; bills are being called medical loss ratio; treatments are being called products; catchment areas are being called covered lives; and mental health is now being called behavioral healthcare—as in the title of this book.

Healthcare is becoming a business and I am becoming a businessman, at least in larger part than ever before. And business ethics are not necessarily the same as medical ethics. Nor are business laws the same as medical laws. The "bottom line" is not the same as "above all, do no harm." While businesses have product liability, managed care companies so far do not seem to be liable for the final treatment decisions made by clinician providers.

It seems that we are now in the process of discovering whether business ethics can fit well enough with medical ethics. Can we have mental healthcare that is both good business like the auto industry, and good for society like education? Is managed care as unethical as many clinicians have claimed, or are we just adapting to cost-effective medical necessity?

HOW WE'LL TRY TO ANSWER THESE ETHICAL QUESTIONS

To discover the emerging answers to these questions, we need to examine some key aspects of the whole process. While many of these questions are relevant for all of healthcare, some unique and peculiar aspects of mental healthcare call for an exclusive focus. Mental health still has a strong stigma associated with it that can separate it from mainstream healthcare. Only in psychiatry did we develop specialized, for-profit hospitals, which brought not only new options for patients but occasional scandalous overuse. Subcontracting for mental healthcare is more common than integration into the rest of healthcare. And many of the primary clinicians in mental healthcare are not physicians.

In the following chapters, we follow an administrator, a manager, a clinician, and other personnel as they idealistically attempt to deal with ethical challenges in managed behavioral healthcare. First, we'll examine what ethical issues might go into forming a managed care system that a prospective patient might enter. From there, we try to use our fictionalized case history as a way to answer the following questions:

- What are the ethical issues in patient triage? It is often no longer possible to simply get a recommendation from a friend and call the friend's favorite therapist for an appointment, so what do we do?
- How should informed consent and confidentiality be handled for patients requiring mental healthcare?
- What are fair financial parameters and responsibility for systems, administrators, clinicians, and even patients?
- How can treatment be planned and performed in an ethical, cost-effective way?
- How should utilization review of that treatment be done and who should do it?
- How much treatment is enough, and who is responsible for the outcomes?
- What can we expect for the future?
- Will we get ethical coding for behavioral healthcare after we get clinical report cards?
- Will business and healthcare mix like oil and water and cause a *Valdez*-like disaster, or like milk and honey to provide us all with enough nourishment?

My goal in each of the following chapters will be to point out the challenges we are all experiencing and suggest some solutions. Since I'm tenured, at least I can discuss these dilemmas without too much fear of the gag rule or recriminations.

We'll introduce other characters to weave an evolving story about how a managed system might develop and struggle with real-life issues. As Jordan Cohen, president of the American Association of Medical Colleges, recently admonished while discussing the fiftieth anniversary of the Nuremberg Doctors Trial, to avoid corruption by power and temptation, healthcare professionals require deep thought, moral struggles, challenging cases, admirable role models, some painful introspection, and extensive study of past dilemmas for context. This book needs the same thought and resources, and I'll also try to add a sense of humor to our serious considerations.

While individual chapters can be read on their own, they're best considered as part of a whole story or a whole system. Just touching different parts of the managed care elephant can be very misleading. Various ethical challenges will be highlighted along the way, with possible solutions. Using an ethical scorecard will be presented as one way to monitor how well we're doing in these areas. However, the ethical challenges are so large that—practically speaking—the real solutions will have to come from all involved in managed behavioral healthcare.

CHAPTER TWO

Establishing
Ethical Principles

❦

One of the chief characteristics of managed care is that it always involves some kind of system. Only a system can provide mechanisms to develop and monitor cost-effective ways of delivering healthcare to large groups of people. In behavioral healthcare, many different kinds of managed care systems have arisen in a kind of marketplace trial-and-error process to see what will be the most successful.

There are systems "carved out" of the rest of healthcare and systems "carved in" to the rest of healthcare. There are systems that just review networks under some insurance plan and there are traditional health maintenance organizations designed to provide everything, as well as a whole range of systems in between. Some behavioral healthcare systems are owned by entrepreneurs, some by hospitals, some by hospital-physician partnerships, some by psychologists or social workers—and there are many other variations. Some are for-profit, some not-for-profit. Some are small mom-and-pop storefronts, while others are heavily traded on Wall Street. The variations almost seem endless. New systems are still starting in some areas of the country, while in other places consolidation and buyouts of massive systems are taking place. As the saying goes, "If you know one managed care company, you know one managed care company."

The ethical challenges for these new systems are enormous. Like anything new, the major challenge is to produce something better without losing anything important in the process. For behavioral healthcare, the central ethical challenge is whether costs can be contained or reduced and at the same time treatment success can be maintained or improved, all the while not ignoring time-tested ethical and legal guidelines.

OUR STORY BEGINS

Adam Wilder was a successful entrepreneur. When the software company he helped develop was bought out by one of the national giants, he made enough on his stock in the company to try something new. He still had his old energy, always there since childhood, when his teachers often called him wild and his high school classmates voted him "Most Energetic." Now that two of his children were also energetic—so energetic they were diagnosed with attention deficit disorder—he realized that he probably had a mild version of the disorder himself. He had found some successful strategies to minimize his problems while using his energy and inventive ways of seeing things, but his kids seemed to need more help than he could give them on his own.

Spurring his current interest in behavioral healthcare was the confusion he encountered in trying to get his children treatment for their more serious attention deficit disorder. He felt his managed care healthcare system gave him the runaround, first telling him that attention deficit disorder might not even be covered under his policy, then later bouncing him between a family practitioner, a pediatrician with special expertise in pediatric neurology, a child psychiatrist, and a mental health family therapist. At least he had found a great private learning disability specialist, but he had to pay for that out of pocket. He thought that as in industry, there should have been a smoother system with clearer guidelines for improvement than he encountered. Now that he had also just turned fifty, he felt he wanted to try something that had more societal need involved.

Evelyn Bloom had been coming to a similar conclusion through a different route. She had been one of those mental health clinicians who try various paths in search of a niche in the field. She had started as a social work caseworker right out of college, not being sure of a career but coming from a family of helpers where she was the oldest child. She worked on an inpatient ward in an inner-city public psychiatric hospital until she burned out, then she took a little time off. After some rest, she decided to become a psychiatrist so as to give herself some expanded tools to help the chronic, seriously disturbed patients she had seen in the hospital. Along the way, she picked up a master's degree in public health to better appreciate the social factors affecting mental illness. As a new psychiatrist, she enjoyed working in a multidisciplinary private practice group. However, as she saw how managed care was affecting the group's business, and as her interest in social factors renewed itself, she tried to get involved with managed care systems. Having recently turned forty, she felt ready for a change and experienced enough to try to take on more of a leadership role.

Adam and Evelyn had known each other a little, both through work and socially. They lived near each other and their children attended the same school, and he had asked her for some informal advice on his children. He in turn had helped educate her and her group on computer programming for their practice.

One thing led to another and they decided to form a partnership to start a new managed behavioral healthcare company before it was too late to get into the market. After all, although political health reform was dead for the time being, marketplace reform was continuing to thrive. The public mental health sector, that sector previously served by state hospitals, academic departments of psychiatry, and community mental health seemed to offer a great deal of opportunity. As states were searching for more cost-effective ways to serve Medicaid patients, they were turning to local and national managed care companies for bids and proposals. The two decided to try their own state—"Central Carolina"—as it hadn't been overrun with managed care yet. They would start slowly and small. They didn't want to be unduly influenced by other investors and the profit motivation, at least at first. As other opportunities became available, they would also pursue those. They set up their company as a not-for-profit corporation. Recognizing that not-for-profit status is not a vow of poverty, however, they made it a basic goal to strive for a 5–10 percent profit on each contract while providing the highest quality of care, so as to have surplus funds to maintain and expand their services. Though excited, they also wondered if they could really achieve these goals in the cutthroat competitive managed care world.

SEARCHING FOR ETHICAL PRINCIPLES

Before embarking on their plan, Evelyn and Adam felt they had to be clear about what values would drive their system, for if they weren't in agreement about the values, major conflict between them would likely be inevitable. They came from different traditions, Evelyn from the medical tradition and Adam from the business tradition. Could these traditions and individuals be compatible? They thought that most other people in their situation would just jump into their arena without any explicit discussion of values or ethics, but they wanted to proceed in the most ethical way possible.

Despite all the potential complexity, they both could see the basic ethical principles involved in rather stark terms: altruism and self-interest. Many ethicists and philosophers, after all, seemed to view altruism and self-interest as the basic principles of moral and ethical life. Although they overlap, one can be used as a guise for the other. How to reconcile these principles seems to pervade human history, including medicine and business. Managed care, it seemed, was calling for a review of how these principles should be applied for the health of our society.

Altruism and Self-Interest

Our two partners thought that a discussion of how their respective traditions handled altruism and self-interest was important. Sensing that business might look worse, Adam asked Evelyn to start. Though she knew some of the general healthcare ethical principles on altruism and self-interest, she asked for some time to review and refresh herself. Sometime later, she presented the following summary to Adam.

The medical tradition has long been concerned with how to balance altruism and self-interest. As far back as the eighteenth century before Christ, the Code of Hammurabi established a payment system for physicians. Moreover, Hammurabi specified that if a patient was harmed, punishment could be severe, including loss of a physician's hands if the patient's life or eyesight was lost as a result of treatment.

Ancient Greece, often viewed as the cradle of modern medicine, produced the medical ethics of Hippocrates. While the Hippocratic Oath is often thought to emphasize altruism, that principle is really only implied in the strictures about what not to do, including to do no harm. Some other precepts seemed to emphasize self-interest, such as the obligations to fellow physicians at the beginning of the oath, which specifies that teachers are to be valued as parents and that the education of future physicians is to be a primary responsibility.

It took the Judeo-Christian tradition to emphasize more of a balance between physician self-interest and the care of others. The medical tradition and Judeo-Christian religious traditions adopted the Jewish theology of the importance of healing through human instruments of God, and added that to Jesus' parable of the Good Samaritan and the duty of charity, to produce a medical ethic with a new balance of altruism and self-interest. Hospitals to serve the needy were an innovation of the early Christian church. The result was supposed to be a physician who could be concerned with financial reward, prestige, and gratitude, but also willing to drop everything else at the call of a patient, and a hospital system that would never turn away those in need.

In modern times, there has been some reappraisal of how traditional medical ethics should be applied. When many institutions were challenged in the 1960s, the medical institutions were also questioned. One result was the application of philosophers, ethicists, and patient representatives to ethical conflicts and dilemmas. A shift from physician paternalism toward patient autonomy ensued. Ethics committees and ethics consultants started to become more standard members of the healthcare team.

A new field, bioethics, became established in the 1970s. Bioethics uses traditional philosophical and ethical principles, applying them to healthcare clinical matters and healthcare systems. Among the many issues and principles covered by bioethics, some of the more important ones for managed behavioral healthcare include:

- *Respect for patient autonomy,* including choice and informed consent
- *Nonmaleficence,* or do no harm
- *Beneficence,* or the moral obligation to help others, including potential conflicts with autonomy
- *Justice,* including allocation of health resources

Codes and Guidelines for Clinicians

As interesting as this summary was to Adam, who saw many differences from the history of how business approached altruism and self-interest, he nevertheless was getting impatient. He wanted to get into action, not spend so much time discussing philosophy and ethics. "So what's this got to do with behavioral healthcare clinicians and managed care specifically?" he asked.

Evelyn was caught a little short, as she enjoyed these ruminations and felt some pride in her field's history. "Please be patient, I'm getting there, and we can't ignore thousands of years of history, can we?" She went on, but turned to behavioral healthcare.

Mental health clinicians, whether they be physicians such as psychiatrists or nonphysicians such as social workers, psychologists, or nurses, have assumed many of the traditional medical ethical guidelines. Her own multidisciplinary history and interaction with other disciplines, she explained, made her realize there were more similarities than differences. Some differences include those that reflect differences in discipline.

For example, the code for psychiatrists is an elaboration of the American Medical Association's Principles of Medical Ethics for all physicians. The psychology code puts some special emphasis on testing and research, while the social work code, adapting the social work paradigm of "person-in-environment," puts some added emphasis on responsibility to society in addition to the individual clients. Some of the mental health disciplines, especially social work, have begun to grapple with the possibility that new ethical guidelines may be needed for managed care.

James Sabin has written a great deal of helpful material on ethical issues in managed behavioral healthcare. He makes a convincing case for how psychiatric ethical principles need to further consider societal needs along the lines set up in the 1993 code of ethics of social workers. He likes to cite a challenging personal example of his own from 1975, when he heard a patient call out, "I have Sabin on the line . . . he used to care about patients . . . now he cares about money!" This anecdote has frequently provoked cogent discussion on how to manage the tensions between the interests of the individual patient and society. Helpful strategies include acknowledging the existence of such conflicts, collaborating with patients to resolve them, and providing competent care. The American Psychiatric Association's Council on Psychiatry and Law has identified four core principles that they felt could be applicable to any healthcare system. These may be summarized as follows:

• The fiduciary principle of placing the patient's interest first should not be supplanted.

• Patients are the ultimate authority for their healthcare decisions, and must have the appropriate information and choice to exercise this authority.

• There must be access to mental healthcare within any particular system.

• The psychiatric profession is responsible for setting standards of care and competence.

"So, are these high-flown ethical principles generally accepted or used anywhere?" Adam asked, getting impatient again.

"Not that I know of," replied Evelyn. "And when you think about it, how can patients always have ultimate authority? The second principle is all very well, but how can it apply to mental health patients who may be psychotic or a danger to others? And, although I'm a psychiatrist, and I think psychiatrists have the broadest biopsychosocial knowledge base of all the disciplines, I'm not sure psychiatrists should always be responsible for setting standards of care and competence. It seems that other disciplines could contribute to that process, and that such responsibility should really cross disciplines and be done by those expert in clinical research."

"It's sure nice to hear someone who doesn't always glibly back their profession when bigger ethical issues are involved," replied Adam. "Do you know whether anybody has attempted to develop ethical principles across all the behavioral healthcare disciplines?"

"Actually, yes," Evelyn replied after some thought. "During my time in the public sector in the 1980s, which was the heyday of community mental health and multidisciplinary teamwork, Eugenio Chavez-Rice, a psychiatrist, set out a general set of ethical principles in mental health in a book chapter he wrote. Like many good ideas, it was ignored, but since managed behavioral healthcare has also come to adopt a multidisciplinary approach, maybe some of these principles should be revived.

"He said we should strive to respond with respect, dignity, and humanism to all patients.

"We should maintain confidentiality unless the patient permits sharing, there is a court order, or there is a life-threatening situation.

"Our primary concern should be the welfare of the patient, and any relationship other than a professional one should be avoided.

"And we should remember that patients have the right to be fully informed of treatment options, and have the right to get second opinions and to refuse treatment unless court ordered."

As Evelyn reconsidered these ethical principles from 1982, they seemed generally applicable to managed care, except for certain omissions and a particular emphasis. How to apply the principles on confidentiality and a patient's right to a second opinion to the utilization review process of managed care seemed unclear, however, as utilization review requires the clinician to share information and obtain a second opinion whether the patient wants it or not. Moreover, these general principles do not address how to resolve financial considerations, especially new managed care financial incentives to limit treatment.

Even emphasizing that the welfare of the patient is of primary concern has been challenged by the ethics of managing limited resources for populations of patients. While the public sector always had limited resources, forcing administrative choices for how much treatment could be given to chronic patients, crisis resolution, children, or those with greater potential for improvement or achievement, there was never the potential to make extra money by limiting services as there is now in capitated mental healthcare. This question of rationing healthcare was especially intriguing to Evelyn due to her experience in the public psychiatric hospital, where she knew treatment possibilities were much more limited than in the fancy new for-profit hospitals.

She recalled another general ethical principle that might apply. The ethical concept of justice, developed by many philosophers and discussed widely in bioethics, would support a decent minimum of healthcare. However, Evelyn realized she was probably getting way beyond her professional knowledge, so she stopped there and wondered if they would need an ethical consultation.

Codes and Guidelines for Businessmen

To Adam, this principle of a decent minimum of essential healthcare made much more sense than equal access to the best healthcare, especially when funding would be limited. After all, the main business ethic he was following was . . . was what? Adam suddenly realized that there were no business codes of ethics he could compare to the ones Evelyn quoted for the health professions.

To be sure, people have been concerned about business ethics for a long time. Over two thousand years ago, Aristotle advised that tradesmen should be excluded from political power. Aristotle's advice was not generally followed, and as far as Adam knew, ethics never became an important concern in business over the centuries. Indeed, greed came to be the password for successful businesses in the 1980s.

Such perceptions of business greed evoked some reflections and admonitions for paying more attention to ethics in business.

Adam knew that in 1983 Douglas Sherwin had written that the purpose of business was to yield profits to the owners and appreciation of capital. Sherwin emphasized that our country has used our founding ideals as the basis for capitalism, to produce economic efficiency in the production and distribution of goods and services that the public desires. His conclusion was that "the means are the ends." Around the same time, Laura Nash had written that there was a wide gap between theoretical ethics and business practice, as illustrated in such jokes as *"Ethics and Business*—the shortest book in the world." When applied business philosophy appeared utopian and sometimes anticapitalistic, business leaders would complain, "You do-gooders are ruining America's ability to compete in the world." Adam also knew that in 1988, Kenneth Blanchard and Norman Vincent Peale—well known for their respective books *The One Minute Manager* and *The Power of Positive Thinking*—developed a short list of "Ethics Check" questions for businesses. They recommended trying to check whether any important business action was ethical by considering whether it was legal, whether it was balanced, and how it made the administrator feel about him- or herself.

"Boy, that sure sounds different from healthcare ethics," interjected Evelyn. "It sounds like business ethics come down to self-interest and comfort."

"You're right, up to a certain point," Adam replied. "Something seems to be changing a little bit, or at least there seems to be more concern about business ethics this last decade. Clarence Walton seemed to call for some broader principles when he described business ethics as how a business should behave toward other organizations, customers, and the environment. Business schools began to incorporate more classes on business ethics. Such classes examined whether there should be limits to profits and compensation, as was the policy of the very successful Ben and Jerry's ice cream company, where the highest-paid employee could earn no more than five times as much as the lowest-paid. Another major ethical deliberation was whether there are other ethical obligations to the community beyond the bottom line for the company. Fareed Zakaria's admonition was to teach business not simply as an acquisitive trade, but as a profession akin to law and medicine where students could see their field as 'noble.'"

"Business as a profession like law and medicine?" Evelyn asked, laughing. "Maybe we should take a little break. Since you just mentioned ice cream, how about some Ben and Jerry's?"

"Great," replied Adam. While he was eating, he thought that not a whole lot of progress had been made by 1996. Yes, individual companies sometimes had their own individual ethical codes, and some companies like the Body Shop, Levi Strauss, and Working Assets had a reputation for focusing on business and employee ethics, but there was still no generally accepted code of business ethics as far as he knew. The corporate system, allowed to flourish to serve the public interest, seemed to be hurting the public interest by drastic downsizing, environmental poisoning, and proliferation of unhealthy products. But at least there were some promising developments. Organizations such as the Josephson Institute of Ethics had emerged to offer training programs for business. Adam was familiar with a publication called *Business Ethics: The Magazine of Socially Responsive Business,* started ten years earlier with a mission statement calling for it to promote ethical business practices by developing a community of business professionals that would model living and working responsibly while creating financially healthy companies. Perhaps, Adam thought, we could adapt their mission statement for our new managed care company. We could also subscribe to the magazine. And the Josephson Institute of Ethics had already been to some of the surrounding communities in North Carolina to introduce their program to emphasize the "six pillars" of good character: trustworthiness, respect, responsibility, caring, fairness, and citizenship. Perhaps "Central Carolina" would also be fertile ground for an ethics-oriented managed care system.

When Adam shared these ideas with Evelyn, she seemed enthusiastic. They were realizing that although at first glance there appeared to be a wide chasm between healthcare ethics and business ethics, given the long tradition of ethical codes in healthcare compared to sporadic attempts to address ethics in business, they could agree on some ethical directions.

After a casual conversation with a hospital administrator about their plans, they discovered one common linkage. Hospitals had always been both businesses and healthcare systems. The American College of Healthcare Executives (ACHE), formerly known as the American College of Hospital Administrators (ACHA), had developed a detailed code of ethics beginning in 1939, six years after the founding of the ACHA. The primary focus has been on administrative healthcare issues, such as conflict of interest, confidential information, resource allocation, and relationship issues with patients, medical staff, and the governing body. Despite covering all these areas, the code failed to resolve the ethical dilemma of when loyalty to the organization should be superseded by duty to the patient. In behavioral healthcare, this dilemma came up in the for-profit psychiatric hospitals that emerged in the 1980s. The ACHE has a process for handling complaints that can result in expulsion, but expulsion only has significance if affiliation with the ACHE has importance to potential employers and colleagues. And whether organizations usually follow these guidelines is questionable.

At the hospital, Adam also noticed the symbol of medicine over the door. "What does the rod-and-snake sign mean, Evelyn?" he asked as they were leaving.

"Interesting you ask that," replied Evelyn, "since the answer suggests another kind of linkage between healthcare and business. Since antiquity, the Aesculapian staff, named for the Greek god of medicine, has served as a symbol of medicine and healing. The symbol is a single serpent coiled around a staff. However, at times the symbol of medicine has been misrepresented as a caduceus, a winged staff with two intertwined serpents. Partially a representation of Hermes, messenger of the gods, this emblem in earlier times was a symbol of commerce and trade."

"So maybe I'll wear a caduceus pin and you can wear an Aesculapian one," Adam laughed.

THE ETHICAL WAY

"So it looks like our professional traditions have some things in common that can give us a solid ethical base from which to begin our company," Evelyn concluded.

"Agreed," Adam responded. "You know, we keep using the phrase 'our company.' Isn't it time to give it a name? While it may seem trivial, a lot of successful businesses spend a lot of money on consultants to come up with an appropriate name for their company. The name can bring up important psychological associations. Let's try to do it ourselves, in the managed care spirit of not spending unnecessary money."

"OK, that sounds like fun—I certainly agree that the name can have psychological associations," Evelyn responded enthusiastically.

"Hmm, how about Garden Healthcare," Adam suggested with a smile. "That name could associate to growth, beauty, and your last name, Dr. Bloom."

Feeling a little flattered, Evelyn paused for a moment, then responded, "Well, Garden Healthcare could also refer to your last name,

Mr. Wilder—some gardens are wilder than others. But don't we want to avoid a wild garden? We want to suggest a system that was carefully planned but flexible."

"OK, I agree that I can use some taming at times," Adam continued. "Hmmm—Evelyn, have you ever been called Eve for short?"

"No," Dr. Bloom replied with a laugh. "So we're not exactly Adam and Eve, but we sure do need to be careful what we do and whom we listen to. Maybe we're taking this garden metaphor too far. After all, don't we just want a name that will indicate we're trying to take the ethical way in managed behavioral healthcare?"

"You've got it, Evelyn!" Adam exclaimed.

"Got what?" Evelyn asked.

"That phrase you used, the ethical way," Adam responded. "Let's just call our company 'The Ethical Way.' Maybe not too subtle, maybe a little grandiose, but it should bring the associations we want."

"That sounds nice," Evelyn agreed. "And we can still keep in mind the garden metaphor, knowing that our endeavor will take hard work, an environment conducive to growth, and a trial-and-error process for developing a healthy product."

"Great," Adam. "We can get started on the stationery right away. How about sharing an apple before we proceed?"

COMMENTARIES ON CHAPTER TWO

It is generally difficult for Americans to accept the notion of a limit to resources, and behavioral health practitioners and consumers are no exception. Even though I am a managed care executive, I'm absolutely convinced that every single American would benefit enormously from psychoanalysis. Aren't you? So why don't we make this an unlimited entitlement for everyone?

The ethics of a social policy, like those of an individual clinician's actions, often have to do with the intellectual ability to grasp larger consequences even when these are not fully understood or valued by professional peers or by patients. When I was visiting India on a Fulbright in 1981, for example, I visited an isolated rural village that, to my surprise, supported a fabulous, state-of-the-art medical center. When we toured the facility (gleaming tile floors, polished medical equipment, Western-educated doctors and nurses explaining everything), I discovered that the disease being treated most often in the center was cholera.

Another interesting aspect of my trip there was that I learned that the village had no sewage system. This, of course, started me thinking about what I would do in that village if I were the Minister of Health. What is the ethical thing to do in an environment of cholera and limited resources: Build and staff this medical center, or build a sewer system? To me, the answer seemed obvious: I'm not a doctor, but it strikes me that the best way to deal with a cholera epidemic is to start with a sewer system and perhaps make the medical center's work largely obsolete—or certainly secondary to this more important, fundamental work.

I've never been able to get that rural medical center out of my head. I think it is a metaphor for how we in the West approach healthcare issues. We feel ethically compelled to treat illnesses and alleviate individual suffering, but rarely do we feel the same tug of conscience to prevent illness in the first place through population-wide interventions. I think we have had the same moral blind spot in our approach to mental illnesses. The best ethical reason I can think of for why we should financially capitate health care providers rather than pay them fee-for-service is that capitation provides a powerful incentive to take the prevention mission seriously, something we have rarely done.

Managed behavioral health care, from my view, is the application of public health concepts, perspectives, technologies, values, and ethics to the issue of mental illness. One of the most important public health perspectives is "population-based planning." The moral struggles so often felt by practitioners when they suddenly find themselves in a managed care environment stems from a background and training that shaped them to focus almost exclusively on the needs of the individual patient before them, and plans evolve accordingly. Indeed, "individualized treatment planning" has taken on the moral aura of a commandment in the mental health professions. There is certainly nothing wrong with this, but what is the clinician's ethical commitment to the larger society as the key person responsible for the caretaking of a scarce resource? If managed care contributes anything ethical to our field, it will tackle the structural supports that often collapse for populations for which we have responsibility, sending individuals to the couch, to the locked unit, and not infrequently to jail. Fee-for-service and cost-based reimbursement certainly hasn't done this. At least under capitation, there is the motive to move interventions much further upstream than we ever have in the past.

It is impossible to talk about ethics without reference to motivation. It is clear to me that there are ethical and unethical managed care companies and practices, just as there are ethical and unethical doctors and hospitals operating in fee-for-service environments. Money, a proxy for most forms of self-interest, is almost always involved in ethical problems. The profit motive has been with us since the very beginnings of healthcare, although if you only pay attention to the mass media, you would think that we managed care executives invented this concept and brought it de novo to our field.

Putting money aside, it is unethical to deny care to anyone, but it *is* ethical for a managed care company to deny access to services that have no value, then suggest (demand) alternatives that do. Capitation is ethical when it gets everyone in the equation thinking about prevention and more economical ways to achieve a good outcome (assuming we can define this). A lot of the concern with ethics derives from our current uncertainties regarding the motives and values of managed care organizations and of the individuals that lead them. These aren't always discoverable in a competitive marketplace—but I hope so.

KEITH DIXON
President and CEO
Vista Behavioral Health Plans

As public-private partnerships in healthcare delivery systems continue to expand, the ethical framework in which practitioners work is now challenged. System reform alters a once-familiar setting and presents new ethical questions. Healthcare reform, particularly as it relates to managed mental healthcare, raises ethical issues when philosophically and fundamentally different public and private sectors merge in mental healthcare delivery systems.

To develop value consensus in the mental health field, it is important to address the concerns of all public and private stakeholders in evolving systems of care. Mutually desirable system goals and outcomes must be determined. Based on this consensus process and agreement on system goals and outcomes, a framework of ethical principles on which these systems should operate can be established.

In looking back historically at the change from institutionalization to community-based services from the 1960s through the 1980s, the public sector recognized the need for a vision and operational values. From these goals, a set of guiding ethical principles called the community support systems (CSS) model emerged. This model focuses on recovery from a holistic perspective employing the strengths of each individual. It emphasizes a continuum of care, from prevention to dealing with the acute phase of an illness to rehabilitation and recovery. The CSS model was instrumental in creating a shift in the way public mental health care was delivered.

In the 1990s, the development of public-private partnerships in the financing and organization of systems of mental healthcare calls upon the mental health field to revisit the ethical framework in the CSS model. These public-sector values in the CSS model should be reviewed in the context of newly developing managed care models and appropriately applied to such systems, keeping in mind the ultimate goal of comprehensive, consumer-centered, quality-driven, cost-effective services that are accessible, appropriate, and responsive to the rights and needs of the individual receiving the service.

In addressing the role of the provider in these new structural arrangements, the ethical principles on which many practitioners base their treatment interventions may be challenged. Prior to managed systems of care, a clinician was able to provide the best treatment he or she determined for that particular consumer. The current shift to managed care tends to focus on population-based interventions via treatment protocols, rather than any individual's needs. Further, mental health specialty referrals may be restricted and procedures for utilization review in managed care systems may constrain the ability of the provider and consumer to design the best plan of care.

To that end, an important issue to address in the development of ethical principles for managed care systems, is how to care for groups of consumers (population-based care) while still maintaining the uniqueness of treatment care plans for any one individual.

There are clear ethical challenges facing us all as providers, public officials, consumers, family members, advocates and businesspeople. Responsibility for the public health and well-being of our citizens must be shared. To attain this goal, the public and private partners in emerging managed mental health systems must engage in a consensus process to establish agreed-upon ethical principles on which to base care.

BERNARD S. ARONS, M.D.
Director
Center for Mental Health Services
Substance Abuse and Mental Health Services Administration

CHAPTER THREE

Forming an Ethical System

Even with the common links they had found, Adam and Evelyn, cofounders and developers of The Ethical Way, felt their traditions were so different that they weren't sure how to proceed. Starting with themselves, how exactly would they work together, and what would be their responsibilities? What would be their official titles? If push came to shove and they disagreed on a major issue, who would have the final say-so? They weren't familiar with other managed behavioral healthcare organizations that had dual leadership. Adam wondered if they should use a consultant.

Evelyn was a little taken aback. "A consultant? Don't we know enough ourselves? Maybe with a little help from our colleagues? And do those consultants really help, anyway? I figure they just get big fees and make superficial suggestions!"

"Not from my experience. I know businesses use consultants much more than medicine. Physicians always seem to feel they know everything. But managed care is so new and in so much flux that an outside, objective perspective could help. And a consultant is a consultant. That is, we don't have to follow the suggestions."

The last point convinced Evelyn, so they went ahead. They rented a small office suite in a building near other healthcare institutions, since they obviously needed a more formal place to start doing business. They hung some of Evelyn's images of healing on the walls and covered the desks with some of Adam's used computer equipment.

They decided on Peter Woods, who was trained both in organizational development and family therapy and who had held a leadership position in a fledgling managed care company until it was bought out. They liked his experience and wanted to have a company that incorporated many of the best aspects of a family. They hoped he could set them on the right path.

STARTING AT THE TOP

Peter Woods affirmed that there would be many advantages to a dual leadership that would represent both clinical and business traditions. Having two leaders from different backgrounds could offer balanced viewpoints and support, though it did also pose a risk of conflict. Administrative and support staff as well as clinical staff would feel represented at the top. Though nodding enthusiastically at the consultant's affirmation of their business marriage, each partner secretly thought that over time it might be possible to learn enough to embody all the necessary qualities of both disciplines as a solo leader. After all, Adam thought, the healthcare ethics might be too big a drag on the business needs; meanwhile, Evelyn felt that Adam would never really accept the overriding importance of her professional values.

Those thoughts led to further discussions about titles and power. Adam asked, "Since everyone in a business has a title, what should ours be?"

"Do we really need formal titles?" Evelyn asked. "Can't we just keep this friendly and informal?"

"Maybe you two could keep it informal between yourselves, but your employees and the other organizations you deal with will need some short-hand way of knowing what each of you do," Peter responded. "Since we're trying to develop a more egalitarian, ethics-based leadership structure, you could use somewhat parallel titles, say for Adam, chief business officer, and for Evelyn, chief healthcare officer. That way we could keep the two ethical systems prominent in everybody's mind." Both nodded in agreement.

"And I assume you two are in agreement about financial responsibility," Peter continued. Here there was some hesitancy in their response. On the one hand, Evelyn felt that since Adam was wealthier, had invested much more in the company, and seemed more concerned about money, he should obviously be responsible. However, she had learned from her prior experience as a provider in managed care that "whoever holds the gold makes the rules." Adam, on the other hand, felt a slight reservation about taking responsibility for the finances. Sure, he had put up 95 percent of $3 million for start-up costs and reserves, so he should be responsible. But while he saw potential for great profits, that wasn't why he decided on this endeavor. As these financial matters were being discussed, Peter saw an opportunity to ask the big leadership question. "Although you two will try to share big decisions, and you'll hopefully make a reasonable profit, if The Ethical Way is in big financial trouble, who is going to pull the plug?"

Both looked at Peter and said, "We'll ask you!"

"But I'm only a consultant," Peter replied, though he felt complimented by the suggestion. "You still have to make the final decision yourselves. However, to answer before the problem may arise, I would suggest that in matters of company survival, Adam have the final decision due to his financial position. This is a business."

Evelyn seemed both relieved and worried.

"I guess that seems appropriate, but for anything with clinical importance, I'll defer to you, Evelyn," Adam eventually responded.

"Ok, let's try it that way," Evelyn agreed. "I trust you, at least for now, especially since I have some important confidential information about you," she continued with a smile, then with a strong twinge of guilt for even thinking about using such confidential healthcare information, even if Adam wasn't really a patient.

"Good," Peter concluded. "I suggest that you hire a lawyer soon to draw up the corporation structure and relationship responsibilities as we've discussed. I can recommend one, if you like." Both agreed.

The consultant was curious why they had early on decided for a 5 to 10 percent profit, since the potential was for more. Adam mentioned that he had recently read that a new Christian-oriented apparel company was committed to limiting their profit margin to 10 to 15 percent, so they decided to have a slightly lower target so as not to let such motivation overwhelm their clinical goals. To further emphasize clinical concerns, they decided to donate anything over 10 percent to financially strapped community organizations like the center for abused women. In continuing to balance clinical and business ethics, they also decided that their initial income should be no more than twice that of the highest-paid clinician. If the company was financially successful over time, they hoped to develop opportunities for part ownership by employees. Adam added, that if need be, he could even delay his salary at first.

Besides these initial financial considerations, Evelyn asked Peter if there were any particular values they should try to espouse as leaders. Remembering something that he thought was said by Mary Kohles, a registered nurse, on the role of leaders in meeting the challenge of providing compassionate and cost-effective healthcare, Peter cited these leadership values as being of particular ethical importance for their stated goals:

- Encourage open communication.
- Be stewards for the well-being of the whole organization.
- Care for the souls of the individuals.
- Model integrity and respect.
- Empower employees.

Evelyn and Adam readily agreed, though they realized that such values were more easily agreed upon than put into action.

Setting Up System Values

After agreeing on those financial parameters, they thought of other possible ways to imbue the organization with appropriate ethics. Although appreciating that ethics codes and guidelines can just be smoke screens or pretenses to obscure unethical practice, they still believed that their use could suggest a certain value system, especially in a new organization.

Besides adopting the mission statement of *Business Ethics,* they adopted the Code of Ethics of the ACHE, which was more specific to healthcare institutions. They especially liked the admonition that members should not invoke any part of the code for selfish reasons. Copies of the mission statement and code were to be given to all new employees.

In considering how to further imbue the organization with high ethical standards, they reviewed the healthcare literature, and didn't find much except a helpful article by Stanley Reiser. Though managed care was curiously absent in Reiser's discussion of the ethics of health-care organizations, the principles still seemed applicable. Reiser stressed that an institution's chosen values must spread throughout the organization. Evelyn and Adam thought that key values for their company, as adapted from Reiser's principles, could be:

- *Humaneness,* or conveying a sense of benevolence and compassion
- *Reciprocal benefit,* or trying to set up a win-win outcome with all relationships
- *Trust,* including valuing those who admit to error
- *Fairness,* or being impartial and nondiscriminatory
- *Dignity,* or showing a respect for all individuals
- *Gratitude,* or appreciation for following the organization's ideal
- *Service,* emphasizing the sanctity of caring for others as above any commercial reward
- *Stewardship,* stressing the need for using resources in the best possible way for the present and future

Among the many notable aspects of these values is how much they overlap the general ethical principles for all mental health clinicians developed by Chavez-Rice, which they had previously discussed. The first principle recommended by Chavez-Rice emphasized responding with respect, dignity, and humanism, and the third principle empha-sized primary service to the medical well-being of the patient.

Although Adam was beginning to have trouble with all these high-falutin healthcare values, worrying that potential profits would plum-met with each principle, he became more enthusiastic when Reiser recommended establishing healthcare objectives and means to accom-plish these objectives. The simple objective they quickly came up with was to provide the best mental healthcare possible within the parameters of their funding basis. The means to accomplish this objective would be establishing certain operations and hiring the best staff possible.

Besides using sound business principles, they felt that a couple of Reiser's recommendations would be especially valuable. One was to establish administrative case rounds where, once a month, key clinical and administrative staff would discuss particular clinical and ethical issues brought up by a real patient case.

Having spent some time in an academic institution, Evelyn wanted to add student rotations and corresponding educational activities. She said to Adam, "I know that most managed behavioral healthcare companies have not been allowing psychiatric residents to see patients. Though they say it's a quality issue, it must be more of a marketing ploy for perceived quality, as if community psychiatrists necessarily produced better treatment results. After all, residents are often more up-to-date about the new medications than older psychiatrists who spent a lot of their career doing psychotherapy, as maturing an experience as doing psychotherapy may be. Besides, we'd only have to pay them half of what we'd pay a psychiatrist, and even with supervision costs added on, we'd come out ahead. Other students, such as social work students and psychology interns, seem to have been used more readily. I think all these students would be cost-effective and spice up any educational activities, such as the administrative case conferences, and keep us all on our toes with their questions."

Saying that they might need some marketing help on this, Adam otherwise agreed, especially since students would be such a small part of their operation.

"You know," Adam continued, "Maybe there is another source of guidelines we could try to adapt to help us find the ethical way. The hospital we visited, that was a Catholic hospital, and they had a booklet lying around called the *Ethical and Religious Directives for Health Care Organizations,* written by the National Conference of Catholic Bishops. Being a somewhat lapsed Catholic myself, I was curious to see what the directives were, and found that many might relate to us."

"Do you remember what they were?" asked Evelyn, who was agnostic.

"Well, here they are, I jotted down some of them in my notebook," Adam replied. "They want to see 'a social responsibility for the public good, with special attention to the poor; respect for human dignity; and professional ethical responsibility in the professional-patient relationship.' They also call for their hospitals to form 'new collaborative relationships' with other healthcare organizations and providers, where they share values such as 'moral analysis, the sanctity of human life, and the promotion of universal access for health services.' There were other directives, including on the beginning of life and dying, but I just skimmed those because they seemed less relevant to us."

"Well, even though I'm not Catholic and neither are many others we'll be working with, those directives you jotted down would certainly seem to be useful for us to follow, especially if we soften them into principles. They certainly coincide a great deal with the professional ethical principles of Dr. Chavez-Rice that we discussed."

"Good," answered Adam. "By the way, I'm sure you've had some exposure to Catholic healthcare institutions. Do they really seem to operate on those principles?"

"I think they really try," Evelyn answered, "but many other things seem to get in the way, such as rigidity, non-Catholic employees and patients, occasional incompetence, and now new financial pressures. And even some stigma issues when it comes to the mentally ill."

Model Systems

With these basic system values in mind, Adam and Evelyn turned to questions of how they would like the system to run from an operational standpoint. How would they maintain their ethical standards? How would they handle ethical transgressions? What protocols would they use for patient care, and why? They agreed that instead of just going off on their own moral inclinations, another way to think about these processes was to look for good ethical models already in existence. Though managed care companies were notorious for the trade secrets and proprietary information of their operations, they did let some information out. There were some published sources to review, and Peter Woods probably had information he could share from his own experience.

Adam and Evelyn certainly did not want to set up a system that produced striking reports of ethical and legal problems like the ones they'd heard of from United Behavioral Systems (UBS), a Rhode Island subsidiary of a major national managed care company. Charges by the state included inappropriate denial of care and improper utilization review. The legal grounding for the charges came from a 1993 state utilization review law that stipulated that no employee or other individual who rendered an adverse decision for a review company could receive financial incentives based upon the number of denials or approvals. The alleged charges included:

• Insufficient grounds for denying treatment in cases where medical necessity seemed to be met

• Not meeting assessment standards for quality of care
• Lack of review by mental health professionals
• Lack of follow-up on problems
• Not providing an appeals process for denied claims

Complaints had come from patients, consumer groups, and psychiatrists. One patient was quoted as saying, "every time you want an appointment, you have to argue with these [UBS] people." A psychiatrist was quoted as saying, "They would tell us 'we'll authorize one [inpatient] day, and then we'll review it.'" The psychiatrist apparently felt comfortable in complaining because he was salaried by a hospital, and the hospital eventually came to support his concerns, cushioning him for any threat of being expelled as a UBS provider.

Adam thought that perhaps the Rhode Island situation didn't reflect UBS in general, as the problem may have just been overzealous local administrators. But after hearing that, Evelyn recalled a related example she had read about in Milwaukee. William Houghton described his surprise about suddenly being taken off the UBS provider list, which was allowed for in their contract in a clause for "termination without cause." Dr. Houghton felt his removal may have come from the recent publication in the *Milwaukee Journal* of an article he'd written that was mildly critical of HMOs in general, but reported that he was never given a reason by UBS. A published response from Mark German, the local UBS executive director, cited "goodness of fit" as the main issue.

Adam and Evelyn decided they wanted to consider only highly regarded managed care systems for any models they could use. Very quickly, the Harvard Community Health Plan (HCHP) popped into everybody's mind. Not only had it had a good reputation for a long time, but much had been written about it.

Harvard is a staff model HMO, formed in 1969, with integrated mental health and general healthcare services. It was said to spend less than 10 percent on profits and administration. Nevertheless, in 1987 there was growing awareness of dissatisfaction with behavioral healthcare services among members, patients, employers, and clinicians. Most interesting to Adam and Evelyn was the process described by Helen Adams, who was a project manager at Harvard at that time, and how that process was used to provide a potentially better system. A planning effort began under the leadership of Harvard's corporate medical director, who also happened to be a psychiatrist. The core planning group consisted of several clinicians—mainly psychiatrists—and some administrative staff. First off, different constituency groups were canvassed, with some feedback that was of particular interest to Adam and Evelyn. Here's what they found out:

- *Members and patients* felt they weren't told enough about their benefits, that having to be referred through a primary care gatekeeper was unnecessary, that they wanted more choice of clinicians and treatment, and more consistency across sites.

- *Employers* felt that mental health coverage could be increased if the benefits were managed better.

- *Clinicians* felt confused over how to balance clinical judgment, costs, and patient satisfaction.

In response to this feedback, management wanted a program that would be easy to understand and simple to administer. They also wanted it to provide better access and improved treatment options for the same available dollars. The dollars seemed sufficient—mental health costs had been rising (14 percent a year) more than other health services and more services were offered than the national norm. In working on the redesign, clinicians admitted that they didn't seem to know how to allocate treatments nor to have a firm sense of what treatments had the best outcomes. The planning group did arrive at a fundamental principle, which was that clinical treatment needs should determine a patient's benefit rather than the other way around.

Evelyn was most interested in the new clinical changes, including the development of an eight-scale Patient Assessment Tool and an expansion of group therapy (including long-term therapy for character pathology) and medical treatments. She was also impressed with the training to implement the changes and the research allocated to study the changes. Adam seemed particularly interested in the co-pay fee structure, which seemed to put some of the responsibility on the patient. This structure had small co-pays for up to eight psychotherapy visits or unlimited medication visits, $35 co-pay for individual therapy and $15 for group therapy for sessions nine through twenty, and complete fee-for-service for over twenty sessions. Both Evelyn and Adam were interested in changes in the delivery system process that the four-year project produced, which included:

- Self-referral to mental healthcare. Contrary to general expectations in the industry, allowing self-referral did not increase utilization.

- Triage by nonclinicians using a standardized instrument with "red flags" for clinician involvement.

- Encouraging informal consultations among the behavioral healthcare clinicians.

Peter Woods suggested that they could adapt the process Harvard used to build a system of their own. This could balance the ethics and values of all the constituents by having the right mix of clinicians and businesspeople working together, with feedback from the payers and insured.

In further pursuing the literature to look for other models, Peter mentioned a description by William Reidy of the then-smaller Community Health Plan (CHP), a not-for-profit staff model HMO based in New England. The development of Community seemed to parallel Harvard, with some additional extensions. With over fifteen years of experience before the article, like Harvard it had emphasized the value of "carve-in" integrated behavioral healthcare benefits and treatments. The values of integration were thought to be coordination of patients with both psychiatric and medical problems, better diagnosis of mental health disorders presenting in primary care settings, quicker help with stress, and reduced administrative costs. Consistent with this orientation, Community emphasized primary care referrals for routine mental health problems, but described the intent of that as a "positive medical screener" to rule out medical problems, rather than a gatekeeper who might try to deflect referrals for financial reasons.

Realizing the traditional HMO staff model was not attractive to purchasers who wanted other behavioral healthcare options, Community set up a review process akin to Harvard's. It also used teams of clinicians and administrators with outreach to payers for feedback. To their surprise, Community management found out that benefit managers knew little about their programs. They then also found out that workplace values were somewhat different from their own. Community had prided itself on medical necessity for treatment and crisis intervention to avoid costly hospitalization. It included the care of more chronic, seriously ill patients. However, the businesses seemed as concerned with any mental health problem, including V diagnostic codes like marital problems, that would reduce work effectiveness. Feedback from patients revealed their general sense that requiring a primary care physician's referral produced an unnecessary and unhelpful delay. As a result of such feedback, Community decided to expand beyond traditional staff model services, to relabel itself as the "premier" healthcare provider group, and to develop a joint employee assistance program.

HIRING AN ETHICAL STAFF

With the basic ethical issues out of the way, Evelyn and Adam felt ready to move on to more specifics. Peter Woods emphasized that hiring the right staff would make all the difference in how well the organization's goals would be met. Although ethical principles would be conveyed and taught throughout the organization, Peter recommended trying to choose people who came in with the desired values, knowing that it is generally harder to teach people ethics than to choose those who already have the right values. Since they hoped that some of their work would be with the public-sector Medicaid population, they also wanted staff with multicultural sensitivity and knowledge who would be able to follow the first healthcare ethical principle of responding with respect, dignity, and humanism.

Middle Management

They decided to start with the next administrative needs that would help them get started. Adam suggested a chief financial officer (CFO) first, while Evelyn wanted a medical director. Peter suggested that since the financial well-being of the company was crucial for its existence, they ought to hire the CFO first. Even though Adam had an accounting background, there were many other things for him to focus on. Adam wondered if Evelyn could supplement the medical director at first until they had a better cash flow. Evelyn agreed and they decided to try to hire a half-time medical director at first. They would try to pay 5 percent above the going rates for such positions to acquire the best quality.

They discussed what else they should consider in hiring these people. They decided to try advertising in business and healthcare publications, and to ask for some experience in traditional healthcare settings so their new administrators would understand the managed care differences. That way these employees would appreciate the ethical implications of traditional fee-for-service, including the tendency to do more and for care to cost more than might be required because the patient's presumed needs always took precedence. They would also appreciate, however, that managed care emphasized cost-effectiveness and saving money, which might possibly lead to undertreatment.

Adam, Evelyn, and Peter weren't sure how to tap into the applicants' values, so Peter suggested an adaptation of the values quiz that Clarence Walton used in his book. They decided to use the following items (true or false, with room for comment):

1. Management is a profession, and managers therefore need a code of ethics just as other professionals—physicians, lawyers, accountants—have codes of ethics.
2. The first things a CEO should demand from other administrators are technical competence and total loyalty.
3. Freud was right in saying that a woman's sense of justice is more subjective and therefore less reliable than a man's.
4. The best reason for building ethical organizations is that it pays off. Good ethics means good profits.

The answers they hoped to find were:

1. True.
2. Generally true, except not total loyalty to someone who does something unethical.
3. Obviously false, though men and women tend to view justice somewhat differently. (With bonus points for describing those differences accurately!)
4. True.

Using these criteria, they were able to hire Buddy Richman as CFO and Barry "The Bear" Grayson, M.D., as part-time medical director. Buddy was told profits weren't the primary goal of The Ethical Way, while Barry was reassured that a medical director wasn't supposed to be a rubber stamp to justify tough medical necessity standards, but rather to be a team member helping develop a sound and cost-effective treatment system.

Clinical Staff

Once these key staff members were on board, Adam and Evelyn turned to consideration of other staff, though choosing clinical staff would have to await the precise kind of contract they would receive. Evelyn knew that clinical staff would need to be comfortable with providing the best treatment under strict financial parameters. Familiarity with brief and intermittent therapies for individuals, families, and groups, as well as expertise in medication, including crisis medication, would be important skills. If clinicians had actual documentation of their own records on cost-effective treatment and patient satisfaction, that would put them in the front of the line for credentialing and hiring. Meanwhile, Adam felt that managerial and support staff would need their particular job skill, but also a sense of value for mental healthcare in general.

Precise numbers of clinical staff would depend on the type of contract, but Evelyn and Adam knew they'd need a multidisciplinary staff that would reflect cost considerations and discipline skills. Psychiatrists would be especially needed for medication expertise, especially with the severely and chronically ill. For hospitalization, they'd look for psychiatrists with a track record of average lengths of stay of less than a week with good results. Master's level therapists—whether social work, pastoral counselors, psychologists, nurses, or marriage and family therapists—would be needed especially to provide psychotherapy. Alcohol and substance abuse counselors would be needed to address those problem areas. Ph.D. psychologists might be needed for testing skills, research skills, and any special psychotherapy skills. Psychiatric nurses would also be needed to deal with common medical problems, as with chronic patients, and to give injections. Social workers with knowledge of free community resources would be especially valuable. For those with strong religious or spiritual needs, especially in the South, pastoral counselors would be needed. With marriage and family therapists, Adam added the caveat that they would need to be good basic therapists, as marital or family problems were often not included as a covered benefit in many managed behavioral healthcare plans. Any potential clinical staff would be canvassed for appreciation of the prior problems with pre–managed care laissez-faire treatment provision, though they didn't have to be completely gung-ho about managed care practices.

Besides considering such a multidisciplinary staff, they agreed on several other hiring principles:

- They would not require certification as the sole criterion for evaluating the quality of the clinician; they would also consider other documentation of clinical skill, including letters of reference and record review.

- They would offer clear information about reimbursement, with no hidden withhold of funds, and with a guarantee similar to whatever guarantee of income the company had.

- They would tie potential bonuses or reduction in future reimbursement to quality of care, financial outcomes, and ethical behavior, not to numbers of denials of care.

- They would offer regular programs for support and to help avoid burnout, especially given the fast pace of managed care work, as well as due process for clinicians who were deemed not to be doing well.

Through interviews and letters of recommendations, information on the applicant's moral values and ethical guidelines would be as valued as the applicant's sensitivity to cost-consciousness. They felt these basic hiring principles would fit most types of managed care contract, including one that brought in Medicaid patients.

Something, or someone, still seemed to be missing as they discussed hiring staff. Evelyn then thought back to other healthcare organizations she had worked for, and being preoccupied with their ethics-based discussion, thought of medical ethicists. Medical ethicists or ethics committees were rarely mentioned as participating in managed care organizations. Perhaps that was due to the emphasis on costs, she thought. While Adam would not agree to a full-time employed ethicist, he did agree to using ethics consultants, who would also offer the advantage of not being influenced by a conflict of interest that might apply if they were employed.

A BUSINESS PLAN

The administrators realized they'd need some sort of a business plan just to get started, although they knew it would need to be limited since they were minimally capitalized, wanted to start slow, and didn't know what sort of contracts they could obtain at first.

They reaffirmed their initial decision to enter the market in Central Carolina, an area of the country where managed care was just beginning to flourish, and where they could avoid cutthroat competition and price cutting just to get market share. Since they valued public service and saw the potential for managed care to make better use of the traditional limits in the public sector, they also wanted to bid on and include public-sector contracts that would allow them to model a one-tier system where patients of any socioeconomic background would receive similar service. They discussed the emerging Medicare market, where they thought the future of managed care and health reform would be played out, but decided to wait until they obtained more experience.

From the financial side, Adam planned on using $1 million to hire the core administrative staff, advertise, and market their company. Buddy, the CFO, thought that this slow but sure start-up approach made fiscal sense. He told them, "The last managed care company I worked for was put together by providers. They didn't do well—had to disband, leaving many treatment providers unpaid and many patients with their treatment hanging. They'd used a legal loophole in their state for provider-owned groups to go at-risk for contracts, since they could in effect function like an insurance company but avoid some of the state licensure requirements that insurance companies have for adequate capitalization."

"So we're different in that we're not mainly provider owned and we seem to have enough capitalization to begin a small contract," Adam replied.

"Agreed," said Buddy, "though we should still be cautious and try to get the less risky contracts at first. Full at-risk capitation could still wipe us out. With the start-up money we have left, it seems we could use up to $100,000 for marketing."

"Any ideas for marketing?" Barry asked.

"Well, I think we need some kind of theme or catchphrase that we can use to distinguish ourselves in the marketplace," Evelyn suggested.

"Those ideas sound great," replied Adam. "Let's hire a part-time marketing person to develop those options and help us get off the ground."

The others nodded in agreement.

"I know someone from my prior job who seemed good with producing effective, educational marketing tools," Adam said. "Her name is Mary Monroe."

"Let's try her," Evelyn responded.

"OK, I'll contact her shortly," Adam said. "Maybe we can start her with designing a brochure we can use both for publicity and as part of any contract proposals we make. Evelyn, how about meeting weekly with whomever we hire to review our progress in this area?"

"Good idea," Evelyn responded. "That way we can also be sure both our clinical and business goals are reflected."

Mary took the job and promptly started to work on the brochure. She loved the phrase The Ethical Way. It reminded her of a song she heard years ago in Texas, where the group "Riders in the Sky" used the phrase The Cowboy Way in a tongue-in-cheek manner to emphasize the right way to be a cowboy. She designed the brochure so that on the front would be a path leading to symbols of health and money. Then below the phrase *The Ethical Way* in bold letters would be:

- Not just The Profit Way
- Not just The Healthy Way
- Not The Wrong Way
- Just The Right Way

"We could go on to say," Mary told them, "that we're not only concerned with saving payers' money, but that we'll provide the best-quality care possible under the circumstances. How we'll try to merge the best of business and behavioral healthcare ethics. How this approach provides extra value."

"Great start, Mary," Adam commented.

After a pause, Barry reflected, "It seems like all these issues focus on the concern that the business ethics of both the payer and the managed care company could produce undertreatment instead of the prior concern of overtreatment. However, if they realize that healthy people and workers are important to the well-being of this country and its business, perhaps even better treatment could emerge."

"That sounds right," Adam agreed. "Let's also emphasize in the brochure that mentally healthy workers will help the success of the businesses and that a mentally healthy population will help our country."

When the brochure was finished, they started to publicize themselves to businesses and governmental systems that might be interested in a cost-effective approach to behavioral healthcare. Adam and Evelyn also began to get in touch with people who might be in a position to help them land a contract.

BUSINESS VERSUS BEHAVIORAL HEALTHCARE ETHICS SCORECARD

After getting The Ethical Way off the ground, Evelyn and Adam felt excited but drained. Adam, who was a betting man and liked to take risks, said, "All this ethical stuff is kind of stuffy and idealistic. Let's have some fun with this, too. How about making this quest into a little game, with a bet on the side. The winner gets to pick the charity of choice for any surplus profits. Since you represent behavioral healthcare ethics and I represent, if you will, business ethics, let's set up an ethical scorecard. Something akin to the report cards that are being done on managed care systems and clinicians."

"Which clinicians seem to hate," replied Evelyn. "But OK, as long as the bet isn't too large. I'm not too big on betting. It doesn't seem to fit my moral code. We'll also need some sort of way to measure results, and how do you ever measure ethics?"

"Well, I was thinking about something like this—" He pulled out a sheet of paper.

- *Both sides win* if the company was around the 50th percentile for quality, 50th percentile for costs of patient care, and 50th percentile for job satisfaction against national norms that were beginning to be studied and published.

- *Business ethics win but healthcare ethics lose* if quality, costs, and job satisfaction all fall below the 10th comparative percentile.

- *Healthcare ethics win but business ethics lose* if quality and costs go above the 90th comparative percentile.

- *Both sides lose* if the quality falls below the 10th comparative percentile and the costs go above the 90th comparative percentile.

After deciding that she understood the game, Evelyn suggested that they might play some exhibition games first before the big game.

There were so many specific ethical challenges they would have to confront along the way—how to triage patients, how to handle informed consent, how to apply confidentiality standards, financial incentives and disincentives, and treatment criteria, how to do utilization review, and when to discharge patients—that they'd need much more discussion if they and their ethical standards were both to win.

So The Ethical Way, after receiving legal advice for such regulations as the federal rule that an HMO serving the Medicaid population must also obtain at least 25 percent commercial enrollers, was ready to open for business. So they advertised, made contacts, and bid, and bid, and bid for business. Nothing happened. They started to wonder if they were trying to be too ethical—and not realistic enough. Then finally. . . .

COMMENTARY ON CHAPTER THREE

Adam and Evelyn have started right in developing a code of ethics for their company. A set of core values, articulated and supported throughout the organization, helps ensure that the vicissitudes and demands of day-to-day operation do not lead the company down a slippery slope of ethical distortion.

Alas, once the values are articulated, they must be applied in the context of savvy business practices and an understanding of the markets. The largest problem is that many of the qualitative features Adam and Evelyn have added to their operating system are not appreciated in the marketplace. The values of the marketplace are a combination of not only the traditions of capitalism (Adam) and providers (Evelyn), but also the consumer movement (traditional American self-reliance) and social welfare (taking care of those unable to help themselves). The interplay of these forces is complex. And in a time of an oversupply of providers and managed care companies and an inability on the part of the purchasers to differentiate between good and not-so-good, the application of provider values in particular becomes difficult.

A 50th-percentile ideal balance between costs, quality, and job satisfaction, for example, is wrong-headed. Midpoint bidders on quality or cost don't win contracts. The marketplace is very demanding, and the ethics and values of purchasers don't often line up with those of vendors; if there is a difference, the buyers usually dominate. The victor is the company that lines up most closely with the buyer's ideal.

For some, the selected vendor must offer the lowest cost with average or better quality. For others, the selected vendor may need the highest quality with costs not dramatically above average. In other cases, it may be possible for a buyer to achieve the 90th percentile on both cost savings and quality: especially if the bidders include organizations that are well established and extremely efficient. Average almost always loses.

If part of the trend in society continues to be taking advantage of an oversupply of behavioral health professionals, pleasing providers with reimbursements also may be contrary to cost-effectiveness and may seriously hurt the company. Since provider costs represent the vast majority of costs in a company, any significant rate differential between The Ethical Way and a competitor will result in a direct pass-through cost. Given that many managed care companies pay only half the fee-for-service rate, providers are unhappy from square one. Paying higher than average fees will decrease that unhappiness, but it will lower the company's pricing score. Again, when cost becomes a less important factor to buyers and when the supply-and-demand equation balances out, provider fees may rise again.

All this is to say that holding fast to your notions of a just world is very hard. At this point in the story, Adam and Evelyn are still idealists, grappling with the theoretical demands of the new business they have begun. The health care marketplace is less flexible than their theories, so they have struggles ahead of them. However, by creating a company imbued throughout with explicit values, they may have the opportunity to sleep better at night.

ALAN J. SHUSTERMAN, Ph.D.
Chairman and CEO
CMG Health

CHAPTER FOUR

Gatekeeping

F inally, Evelyn Bloom and Adam Wilder, the clinical
and business partners of The Ethical Way, landed a managed care contract. Well, a small subcontract. Their organizational consultant, Peter
Woods, had put in a good word for them with the owners of another
managed care company, which had obtained a general healthcare case
management contract for 100,000 people from an insurance company.
Actually, the other managed care company was a subsidiary of the
insurance company, so it had an inside track to get the contract—a
two-year administrative services only (ASO) contract to provide a gatekeeping process for how patients could get care, to develop a network
of clinical providers, and to review treatment for medical necessity.

Now the other managed care company wanted to subcontract the
behavioral healthcare portion in a carve-out to a company like The
Ethical Way, which they hoped would have better expertise in this
specialized—and potentially costly—area. The Ethical Way's competitive bid was for 25 cents per member per month to provide the ASO
for behavioral healthcare needs. The expectations were that satisfactory treatment would be provided to the mainly blue-collar population while keeping total behavioral healthcare costs below $4 per

member per month. Although this money only covered specialist behavioral healthcare, and not that provided by primary care physicians, another expectation was that mental health costs for primary care physicians would not balloon. How to perform all these processes was up to The Ethical Way.

"So, first things first," Adam said, itching to get going.

"And we've got so much money, what—" Evelyn began.

"Three hundred thousand, Evelyn," Adam impatiently finished for her.

"OK, OK," continued Evelyn with some irritation. "So it's clear we need to use some of the money to set up a gatekeeping process for behavioral healthcare needs, use some of the money to set up a network of clinical providers, and some of the money to hire utilization reviewers to review any proposed treatment for appropriateness. And we don't use the money to pay clinicians, but we can set the rates of payment that will come out of the budget of the managed care company with which we have our subcontract."

"Right," Adam responded. "We just need to try to make sure that they don't end up paying over $4 per member per month for behavioral healthcare providers. And not have a balloon in the mental health costs of behavioral healthcare provided by primary care physicians.

"So our CFO [Buddy Richman] and I worked out a preliminary budget, and we came up with the following:

"One. Hire a contract administrator to work with our medical director [Barry "The Bear" Grayson] to set up the gatekeeping process and develop the network, at $75,000 a year (with fringe benefits).

"Two. Hire two utilization reviewers to monitor the recommendations of the gatekeepers and the treatment performed by the providers, at $55,000 each (with fringe benefits). The reviewers would report to the medical director, who would meet them weekly, review all their written decisions on authorization, and respond to any appeals made by clinicians or patients.

"Three. Develop a management information system that could process and document who is doing what type of authorized treatment, at $100,000 to establish. Of course, this would be an expense that could also be used for later contracts, though the computer system would likely need future adjustments and upgrading."

"So that totals $285,000, for a potential profit of $15,000 or 5 percent," added Evelyn with a smile.

"Not exactly," Adam quickly retorted. "We'll need three more offices, connected to each other in a suite, but I thought we'd take that out of our start-up costs."

After using some of their three months' preparation time to hire the new staff and get the computer system in place, Evelyn and Adam had a meeting to further discuss how they wanted to do the gate-keeping process.

GATEKEEPING CHALLENGES

Adam, as usual, began. "First, prospective patients have to get in the door. Or, in managed care terminology, get through the gate, as in gatekeeping. And I sure don't want any obstacles for that. People shouldn't get a runaround like I did when I wanted to get help for my sons' attention deficit disorder. Like I had previously mentioned, let's just keep the gate wide open."

"But won't there be different clinical and financial outcomes depending on who minds the gates?" Evelyn said. "If we want to follow some of our basic behavioral healthcare ethical standards—show respect, give patients some choice, keep confidentiality, focus on the patients' best interests, and all the while watch our costs—don't we need gates that not only swing open easily, but that also lead to the right clinical places and that shut securely behind soundproofed and modestly comfortable offices staffed by clinicians expert in cost-effective techniques? Let's bring in Barry to further discuss how we want to do this gatekeeping process."

"Great," Adam agreed. "We'll need someone who has broad clinical knowledge, is comfortable with risks, is respected, has a commanding presence, and can be tough enough to just say no at times."

Barry "The Bear" Grayson, whom they had recently hired half-time as medical director, had been a popular medical director in managed care systems since he tended not to see issues in terms of just black or white, and he certainly could be tough enough to instill a little fear when necessary. What had gotten him into difficulty at times—and contributed as much to his nickname as his large size—was his gruffness, which could cause public relations problems for the companies. And, if there was anything that managed care companies wanted to avoid, a bad image was high on the list. Evelyn and Adam got a first-hand look at The Bear's gruffness when they sat down with him to discuss the gatekeeping process and whether to keep the door open wide.

"You two are sure nice. Too nice," he said a little sarcastically. "Let's have some gates that are a little harder to open and that lead to some secret passageways. If too many people come for help, and especially if they go to the wrong places, their treatment will suffer, the costs will escalate, and you'll lose your contract."

"You've got a point," Evelyn replied. "But let's not be so secret. That's not the kind of ethical system we want, is it? We want both appropriate help and appropriate profit."

"You may want that, but if you want me I say we have to be a little secretive, or at least controlling of our information and operational processes," the Bear quickly retorted.

"Maybe we're just arguing semantics here," Adam suggested. "Barry, you don't really want secrets, do you? Just the right way to guide patients. And I'm sure you can help us with the right paths."

The Bear softened. As he aged, he was becoming more like a Teddy bear, and that, along with his legendary knowledge of treatment research, was why Evelyn and Adam had decided to take a chance on him, though they would try to keep him behind the scenes as much as possible.

WHO SHOULD SERVE

"Well," Evelyn continued, "we sure have a lot of possibilities for prospective patients who could enter our system. There seems to be no clear consensus in managed care and no research that adequately compares the options. Some of the many possibilities are:

> "*Primary care physicians* as the sole gatekeepers, who will then decide whether to provide treatment themselves or refer to a behavioral healthcare clinician
>
> "*Telephone gatekeepers*—either variously trained staff or a computer system
>
> "*Behavioral healthcare gatekeepers,* who could be representatives of any discipline
>
> "*Patient gatekeepers,* where prospective patients could just refer themselves for treatment to anyone of their choice."

"Maybe we should just toss the possibilities up in the air and try one," Adam said with some seriousness.

The Bear countered, "There is some literature out there that will help us to distinguish the pros and cons of these options for cost-effective patient care. Since primary care physicians have often been given the gatekeeper responsibility and I myself had some family practice training before I went into psychiatry, let's start there."

Primary Care Gatekeepers

Even though he had some training in family practice, or maybe because of it, Barry was very much against primary care physicians being designated as the primary or sole gatekeepers because most do not often recognize mental health problems as such. He started to reel off example after example:

"Whose panic is the problem? I can't tell you how many cases I've seen or reviewed where someone comes in with a history of intermittent intense anxiety, vague chest pain, shortness of breath, and a fear of dying. More often than not the patient gets sent for thousands of dollars' worth of cardiac workup instead of treatment of panic disorder. Maybe the physician is also panicking.

"You don't have to feel depressed to be depressed. Then there are all the cases—especially in patients from minority ethnic groups—of lethargy, poor sleep, weight loss, vague somatic complaints, and hopeless feelings that get worked up for cancer or an endocrine disorder, but nobody asks the patient about any major personal losses suffered right before the symptoms that might suggest a diagnosis of a depressive disorder.

"It's not just growing pains. Then there are all the children and adolescents who are thought to have normal developmental problems, but really have early signs of conduct disorders, anxiety disorders, or even bipolar disorder."

The Bear sighed. "I could go on and on, though of course there are exceptions. And there's all kinds of research to back up my experience. Going back over fifty years, Nick Cummings and Mike Sayama reported that Kaiser Permanente HMO in northern California found that over 50 percent of physician visits were by patients who had some sort of undiagnosed mental health disorder. Fifty years later, it looks like not much has changed, as reported by Arline Kaplan, Sheila Fifer, Barry Blackwell, and others. To make matters worse, depressive disorders in patients in some prepaid plans seem to be even less recognized by primary care physicians than depression in patients in fee-for-service plans! Then if you add on that while primary care physicians have been trained to make referrals to specialists, they have not been trained to try to keep patients away from specialists in a gate-keeping function. Nor have they generally received courses in economic issues in medicine."

"So we at least have an ethical problem of competence if we designate primary care physicians as gatekeepers, don't we?" was Evelyn's somewhat rhetorical question. "Any other ethical problems you can see, Barry?"

"Isn't that enough?" The Bear snapped.

"Well, actually I think there are some nonclinical business issues for us to consider, too," interjected Adam. "Let's look at the possible financial influences. The financial parameters and influences on primary care physicians may vary depending on how much responsibility they have for behavioral healthcare costs. In a completely integrated system where behavioral healthcare is as much a part of the whole treatment system as any other medical specialty, the primary care physician is often given responsibility—and sometimes bonuses—for keeping overall costs down by controlling referrals to specialist care like behavioral. In that kind of system, the primary care physicians could be financially motivated to do more of the behavioral health-care themselves, along with being the gatekeepers, as that could keep overall costs down. As we've discussed, that may pose ethical problems as it could compromise proper early recognition and treatment of behavioral healthcare problems.

"So, in a carve-out behavioral healthcare situation like ours, where we are responsible for developing cost-effective behavioral healthcare provided by mental health providers, the primary care physician may be financially influenced to recognize as many mental health problems as possible, and then refer to the carve-out system. As we've seen, that may be good from a patient care standpoint. And it should be cheaper since the patients will likely get cost-effective brief behavioral healthcare instead of unnecessary and expensive medical testing."

"But the problem of poor recognition of behavioral problems by primary care physicians remains," Evelyn added. "So, before we decide not to use primary care physicians as gatekeepers, are there any solutions to these ethical problems?"

"Possibly," replied a calmer Barry. "One way is through better education. Another is through diagnostic manuals geared to the way patients present to primary care physicians rather than to the way mental health specialists see them. Hopefully, the new diagnostic manual that the American Psychiatric Association put together especially for primary care physicians, *The Diagnostic and Statistical Manual of Mental Disorders—Primary Care Version,* will make a difference. It uses symptom groupings and algorithms to expedite the diagnostic process, and includes descriptions of psychosocial problems other than mental disorders that are commonly seen by primary care physicians.

"Then there are system solutions. Primary care physicians could function cost-effectively within a capitated system by having precise and timely communication with a small panel of consultants, with an initial maximum of two consultant assessment visits. If we can accomplish some of these improvements, that would help satisfy the ethical guideline of trying to meet patient choice, since many more patients with mental health problems still prefer to go to primary care physicians before they would go to mental health clinicians."

Telephone Gatekeepers

"Since it looks doubtful that the primary care physician as gatekeeper will meet our ethical expectations any time soon, at least to be the sole gatekeeper, how about something much more simple, yet technologically advanced?" suggested Adam, calling on his software background.

"Do you mean those 800 numbers answered by high school graduates? They just use a person's zip code to give three clinical options." The Bear growled. "If prospective patients ask for more options, they may be told there is no such list. I mean—"

"Wait a minute, wait a minute," Adam interrupted. "We wouldn't do that. If we use 800 numbers, we'd need to select carefully trained mental health personnel, who would be given guidelines on confidentiality, and have more expert backup. But beyond that, how about me designing a fancy new computer hookup that can ask standardized diagnostic questions over the phone?"

"Won't that be too costly to set up?" retorted The Bear. "Especially since we'll really need a video component to see nonverbal signs."

"How often is the nonverbal information so crucial?" Adam asked.

"Often enough," the Bear countered. "You might miss some of the inappropriate responses of a schizophrenic patient or the tense body language of someone ready to explode. Missing such clues could lead to missed early intervention, decompensation, and higher costs."

"Well, this doesn't sound too cost-effective either," Evelyn concluded. "Without effective gatekeeping, long-term costs will rise due to worsening of symptoms or ineffective treatment."

Adam reluctantly agreed to give up on telephone gatekeepers for the present.

Mental Health Clinician Gatekeepers

"So it looks like our gatekeeper is coming down to a mental health clinician," continued Evelyn. "I mean, given the known limitations of primary care physicians and telephone triagers, can we assume that in-person triage by a mental health clinician would be the most ethical, at least in terms of the patient's best clinical interests? Certainly that would be true if basic diagnostic accuracy was the sole ethical issue. However, if costs are also a consideration, not only is there as yet no documented evidence that mental health clinicians are more cost-effective at triage, there are also lingering questions whether they may increase expenses."

"Mental health clinicians who are oriented to only the best or ideal treatment may tend to triage patients to clinicians and treatments that will not fit into the overall cost considerations of the individual patient's benefits or the system as a whole. For instance, a capitated system at today's prices would likely go bankrupt before being able to accommodate many psychoanalyses, despite whatever justification can be given for psychoanalysis being the best treatment available."

The Bear, referring again to the literature, added that, amazingly enough, he knew of no available research to answer which mental health discipline is likely to do the most cost-effective triage. That is, it remains unclear whether psychiatrists, psychologists, social workers, psychiatric nurses, or even trained paraprofessionals should do the first level of triage. "I think there are unresolved ethical questions about each, which can be summarized as:

> "*Psychiatrists*—they're arguably the broadest trained and can presumably better rule out any medical disorder, but how often are their special diagnostic skills needed and would they turn out to be too expensive if they were the exclusive first line of triage?
>
> "*Psychologists*—they have the advantage of training in the use of psychological testing to supplement diagnostic interviewing, but

they are not medically trained and traditional psychological testing is more extensive and expensive than may be relevant for routine triage.

"*Social workers*—they may be the cheapest discipline. They have been traditionally used for triage in community mental health centers, and usually have the best knowledge of community resources, but they also are not medically trained and generally have less training than any other discipline in making psychiatric diagnoses.

"*Other kinds of therapists, like marriage and family therapists*—they'd be as cheap as social workers, or cheaper, but they may not have as much knowledge of how to use inexpensive community resources such as self-help groups.

"*Paraprofessionals*—they'd have the lowest up-front costs, but they don't have any standardized training, ethical code, or licensure, so their skills and conduct are liable to vary widely."

Evelyn then remembered about the team triage she was part of as a social worker in the public sector. She knew that in this structure, a nonpsychiatrist often would be the first contact and do the initial intake, with a psychiatrist available for backup whenever clinical judgment or designated red flags indicated need for another perspective. So she suggested that maybe a designated team or teams could be the gatekeeper.

"If you want," growled The Bear. "It sounds nice, fairly cheap, with many perspectives available. But here too, we have no comparative data as to success. We do know that responsibility for the patient often falls through the cracks in teams. There are no ethical guidelines or legal regulations for mental health teams that I know of."

"So is there anything you think we can do to deal with the ethical problems of mental health teams being the gatekeeper?" queried Adam, getting ever more impatient for a simple solution so they could get on with the company's real work.

"Sure," said The Bear. "Any clinical staff we hire or use in the surrounding network should be assessed for their knowledge of the strengths and weaknesses of their own disciplinary training and costs, and not be tempted to do more or less than they are capable of. That is, we can't have anybody feel that they can diagnose anybody conclusively if they just use the psychiatric diagnostic cookbook. Just because some psychologists think they are ready to get prescription privileges doesn't mean they also have the basic knowledge to be able to rule out possible medical illnesses masquerading as behavioral symptoms. And psychiatrists, just because they have the most comprehensive training and are still paid at least a little more, shouldn't think they know it all and need to at least eyeball every new patient. Though we psychiatrists espouse the biopsychosocial model, we're notoriously weak on the social part, including knowledge about cost-effective community resources."

"Are there any characteristics you think any mental health clinician should have if they want to do gatekeeping?" asked Evelyn.

"Yes, that's an important question since this is such an important function, and not for everybody," answered Barry. "I'd say the ability to establish quick rapport, an active style, comfort with limited information, and a broad knowledge base are all important."

"Well, about the only discipline you haven't mentioned is psychiatric nurses," Adam added with a hint of challenge.

Taken aback a little, The Bear retreated to consider that possibility. After all, psychiatric nurses had both medical and behavioral health-care knowledge, and even psychodynamics if they were trained along those lines. Some had limited prescriptive privileges. But their numbers were small. . . .

Patient Self-Referral Gatekeeping

"So we've gone through the primary care gatekeeper, the telephone gatekeeper, and just now the various mental health gatekeepers and all seem to have some potential ethical benefits and problems," Adam continued. "So why don't we just allow prospective patients to open the gate themselves and go wherever they want whenever they want? We all know that some managed care systems permit bypass of any designated gatekeeping system and allow the patient to self-refer to any clinician within the network, or out of the network if a point-of-service option is available. Having to go to a certain gatekeeper must be really confusing for the public. People don't have to do that when they go to a lawyer, or buy a car, or rent an apartment."

"True," replied Evelyn. "But while that option certainly supports the bioethical principle of patient autonomy and may enhance continuity of care, it may cause other ethical concerns. We know very well that only a small percentage of those with mental disorders seek treatment, so leaving the request for behavioral healthcare up to the patient more often than not seems to lead to no request. Conceivably, much medically necessary treatment goes unrequested."

Those comments snapped The Bear out of his reverie about psychiatric nurses, and sensing a kill, he snarled, "There goes your old bleeding social worker heart, Dr. Bloom. We'll all go starving if we try to bring everyone who needs help in to get help. And does the payer really want that?"

Evelyn had the urge to fire The Bear right then and there. But she also realized he had a point, both about her and the system. "I don't know if the payer wants that. Maybe they should want that. We can try to find out. And maybe we can educate them as to the benefits of some primary preventive services, which was one of the original goals of health maintenance organizations, but apparently got lost in the competitive fury over costs. If business companies want to save medical costs and workplace costs in the process, then more member education, primary preventive services, and outreach may be ethically indicated. We could even suggest instituting a mental health checkup where mental well-being was checked at various developmental times, say, along with immunizations or school physicals for children and along with physical checkups for adults. Well-trained nurses should be able to do these cost-effectively to check for normal psychological development or early signs of undue trauma, depression, anxiety, and substance abuse."

"And speaking of education," Evelyn continued, "the public should also be educated as to the limitations of self-referral, especially via a recommendation by a friend. Even though friends may have similar interests or tastes, the main indication that a diagnosis or treatment would turn out to be similar would be biological commonality rather than social commonality."

Ever interested in sound research, Barry started to wonder about the ethical and clinical implications of having the gatekeeper also become the treater or to separate the functions. Having a triager become the treater offers continuity of care and the potential for a quicker therapeutic alliance, but may reduce patient choice and provide temptation to provide unnecessary treatment. Separating the functions might offer the ethical advantages of reducing conflict of interest and providing a valuable second perspective, but also cause delays getting treatment started. He felt this question had special importance to certain patients, especially those with borderline personality disorders. He remembered so many likely borderline patients storming out after being told after the initial evaluation that they were being referred to another thera- pist in the clinic. "Why? Don't you like me? Don't I pay enough?" The hypersensitivity of patients with borderline traits or disorder, and their tendency to split teams, would likely cause havoc with split clinical functions. Of course, he smiled to himself, clinicians often liked the option of referring borderlines—such patients were taxing to treat.

Making a Choice

Adam, ever ready to move on, then broke the silence, "Enough of these deliberations, as interesting as they may be. What are we going to do? I have been convinced by all this information that telephone triage is not the way to go at this time, nor is patients' self-referral to whoever they want. I probably should defer to you here, Evelyn, because the clinical considerations are paramount."

"Thanks, Adam," Evelyn responded. "And despite the lack of con- clusive research to guide us, we do have to decide. I'd say let's use master's level clinicians as our key gatekeepers, and initially choose them based on the characteristics Barry just recommended. We'll also insist that a psychiatrist be on site for backup assessment whenever necessary."

"I'm comforted that you agree that the gatekeepers should be able to establish quick rapport, be comfortable with limited information, and have a broad knowledge base, all of which I'll look for in choosing them," Barry added. "I wonder, though, if we can't add a little pilot research project to help verify whether we're making the right decision."

"Please explain more," Adam said.

"Well, maybe we can still do some comparative research about all these gatekeeper possibilities. Perhaps, say, every tenth or every twen- tieth patient that calls for behavioral healthcare can be randomly referred to other gatekeeping mechanisms, then we can study the out- comes after a year or two. I suggest we develop a small contract with a Central Carolina medical school department of psychiatry for some objective research help. If we just do it ourselves, it can look like eth- ical conflict of interest.

"Sounds like a good idea, Barry," Evelyn responded. "Let's try to do it. Maybe we could discover a better ethical way for entering behav- ioral healthcare. Perhaps we can identify other clinician characteris- tics that improve gatekeeping regardless of discipline.

"OK, enough," Adam concluded. "We know how we're going to do gatekeeping, but gatekeeping for what? In other words, what criteria will our gatekeepers use to make their decisions?"

MEDICAL NECESSITY

Whatever gate is used for prospective patients, managed care has brought about the extensive use of a special kind of passcard to get through. That passcard is so-called medical necessity. All gatekeeping functions in managed care seem to have as their goal to determine whether any behavioral healthcare is medically necessary, for unless it is medically necessary, authorization for payment of treatment will not be forthcoming. "So, whoever does the gatekeeping, even patients themselves, will have to know what we mean by medical necessity," Evelyn emphasized.

Evelyn vaguely remembered that medical necessity was a term that was used at times in the pre–managed care days. But its importance was so limited that it had not been mentioned in any of the traditional healthcare or behavioral healthcare ethics codes of that time. However, in managed care it had become ubiquitous; it was a major source of ethical controversy and conflict between clinicians and managed care companies. Evelyn could roll the typical examples off the top of her head:

"Does somebody who has been a little unhappy most of his or her life, but who functions adequately, qualify as needing medically necessary treatment under insurance coverage? Prozac seems to help some of these. Or is this just a common problem of living, the luck of the draw, that should be paid out-of-pocket for self-improvement?

"While medication for severe mood swings in bipolar patients may commonly be thought to fit medical necessity criteria, what about the ensuing marital therapy that may be desired to repair the damage of the mood swings?

"What about the medical necessity of sociopaths, who cause enormous societal problems but are unlikely to succeed in treatment?

"Is gender reassignment surgery medically necessary to help patients thought to have transsexual disorders?

"Is psychotherapy medically necessary for victims of known trauma such as sexual abuse, even though they seem to be happy and adjusting well at the time?

"When is hospitalization medically necessary for suicidal ideation? When is it medically necessary for cocaine intoxication? For command hallucinations associated with a psychotic depression? When a patient has an imminently terminal medical disease?"

Evelyn could go on and on. She wondered what Barry thought, given all his research knowledge. "Barry, how would you define medical necessity for us?"

Definition of Medical Necessity

"I'm glad you asked me, since it seems like it is often administrators who define medical necessity, not necessarily medical clinicians, though medical directors may give their stamp of approval anyway. From my knowledge and reading, it appears that individual companies may vary quite a bit in their definitions."

"They probably do. But from the business standpoint, they'll claim so-called proprietary information as a reason not to share those definitions, unless state utilization review laws require them to do so," Adam added. "The big business concern is whether a broad definition of medical necessity will be a bottomless pit and be too costly."

"If all this is so secret and vague, what criteria should we use? Or should we just throw out medical necessity altogether?" asked Evelyn.

"No, of course we shouldn't get rid of medical necessity," growled The Bear. "Every decision for authorization of payment will be even more subjective then. There is some literature we can use that I'm familiar with. William Glazer has argued for an approach to medical necessity that considers the provider, the disease, and the treatment. The provider need not be a medical clinician, but would need to be supervised by a physician, though how much supervision is left unclear. A medically necessary disease would be any DSM-IV disorder, not to include V-codes ("Additional Conditions That May be a Focus of Clinical Attention") like grief. To be medically necessary, treatment would need to be appropriate and effective. Appropriateness refers to level of care, or 'the least restrictive environment.' Effectiveness refers to likely success, so that medication is often offered earlier to meet medical necessity than the uncertainties of the various psychotherapies."

"All this still seems pretty vague and subjective," Evelyn responded. "Isn't there anything better for us to use?"

The Bear bristled and retorted, "Sure. James Sabin and Norman Daniels published a wonderful, scholarly discussion of medical necessity in mental health practice. Their conclusion is that we should use the normal function model that accepts that the central purpose of behavioral healthcare coverage should be restricted to disadvantages caused by diagnosable disease. That is, people who are unable to function normally or adequately in society due to a diagnosable mental disorder should fit medical necessity and be covered by health insurance. This model would best fit practical societal needs for medical necessity."

"That sounds fair, but if we let clinicians know this criterion, won't they manipulate their information to fit?" Adam asked. "I remember reading somewhere that up to 70 percent of physicians would deceive insurers if they felt insurance criteria were unfair. How ethical is that?"

"Well, Sabin and Daniels weren't naive," countered The Bear. "They recommended authorization for at least three to six evaluative sessions so that the diagnostic determination would be more certain and allow time for referral to other alternatives for help if indicated. That way, the clinician could still feel like a caregiver rather than just an in-or-out gatekeeper."

"Three to six sessions for an evaluation!" Adam exclaimed. "Three to six hours? You're sure being generous with our time and money. I don't think hardly any managed care companies approach approving that much evaluation."

"So what?" The Bear snapped back. "Does that make it right?"

"No," replied Adam, "but if we expect to meet the national average of six to eight outpatient sessions, then three are already gone. And I suppose children would need even more since their situation is often more complicated."

"I also wonder about the emphasis on diagnosis—in the past, research has indicated that psychiatric diagnosis is a poor indicator of resource need or use," Evelyn added.

"OK. You both know what I'm going to say," Adam said. "It's time to decide, at least for the time being. And I don't think it would be ethical for me to try to twist your arms to get approval for a definition of medical necessity that you didn't support. I do believe that we all already agree that medical necessity is potentially an ethically valid business and healthcare concept. For business purposes, it could save money by reducing questionable treatment. For healthcare ethics, it potentially is one solution to the rationing problem by emphasizing the more significant behavioral problems. The ethical dilemma is where to draw the line for medical necessity."

"Yes, it is," Evelyn responded. "Barry, as medical director, the decision is yours."

"OK, thanks," said Barry. "I'd base ours on the Sabin and Daniels definition:

"One: a diagnosed DSM-IV Axis I or II disorder, with the required symptoms documented on the treatment plan.

"Two: impaired social functioning as a presumed consequence of the disorder.

"Three: treatment that is available to help, and that can be justified by professional literature and monitoring of effectiveness."

A Case Example

Shortly after their case management contract started, a case came to their attention at the regular monthly conference they had decided to use when they were forming The Ethical Way. Though an unusual activity for a managed care company, these conferences allowed them to get a closer look at ethical issues, and were a nice tie-in to their relationship with the nearby department of psychiatry and behavioral sciences, which was also sending students to them to see patients and learn about managed care.

This case centered around the question of medical necessity. The presenter was Ricky Manley, one of the utilization reviewers hired for the contract. She started, "This is a case of possible attention deficit disorder (ADD)."

"Great," interrupted Adam. "I'm glad we're paying attention to ADD. I hope we do better than the experience I had with my kids."

"This is a case of possible attention deficit disorder in a thirty-five-year-old woman," Ricky continued. "She self-referred after reading a newspaper article on attention deficit disorder in adults, and thought it fit her. She called her primary care physician, who was comfortable evaluating ADD in children and prescribing Ritalin, but didn't know what to do here. So he called one of our gatekeepers, who did know a couple of psychiatrists who supposedly had some expertise in this area."

"That's good," said Barry, "even though research is indicating that large numbers of children with ADD have symptoms persisting into adulthood, it has not become a standard diagnosis. Psychological tests are usually very expensive and often inconclusive, and in some places it's becoming a faddish diagnosis to explain everything from substance abuse to laziness. So this kind of a case often doesn't quite fit the medical necessity criteria we developed, so we need to have some flexibility in coming to a diagnosis. On top of all of this, some of the medications that can help are abusable if they get into the wrong hands."

"So we could have a scandal on our hands if those medications turn out to be abused or sold on the street," commented Adam with some concern.

Meanwhile, Ricky continued. "So the patient was evaluated, and we gave two sessions with a network psychiatrist. Usually we give one session, but two seemed necessary to have enough time to get feedback from significant others, including the mother. The mother filled out the brief WUCS scale, which indicated likely ADD. She reported that her child had not really been hyperactive or impulsive, in her terms, but effervescent and tomboyish. The girl's grades were spotty, especially in subjects requiring a lot of reading, and she had trouble sustaining concentration. Her charming personality and other skills helped her develop a business career through sales. But relationships were tempestuous, and she turned more to alcohol and sedatives to calm herself. As she moved into upper management at work, she started to have trouble reading complicated proposals, acting calmly, and being able to delay decisions."

"Sounds like a normal variation to me," a student clinician volunteered.

"Perhaps," responded Evelyn. "But she may have ADD, her functioning is worsening, and there are some treatments that may help. All of that suggests likely medical necessity."

"And what does the clinician propose with his treatment plan?" Adam was interested in knowing, as he even wondered if it would apply to himself.

"A trial of Ritalin, a referral to a therapist he knows for some supportive therapy, and if we know of one, a learning disabilities specialist for adults to help with the reading problems," Ricky answered. "I wasn't sure if all of that was medically necessary at first."

"I doubt it," chimed in The Bear. "Though medication is worth a try, and tentative results should be available quickly, the psychiatrist should be able to incorporate a little supportive therapy into the medication checks, for which we'll pay for twenty minutes instead of fifteen. As to the learning disabilities specialist, are there any available in our network?"

"I'm not sure," responded Evelyn, "but I'm not even sure if teachers would be considered to be providers under her insurance contract. Let's start with the medication and go from there."

BUSINESS VERSUS BEHAVIORAL HEALTHCARE ETHICS SCORECARD

As the administrative case rounds ended, Evelyn and Adam began chatting. "Very interesting," opined Adam. "I sure am learning a lot about the ethical challenges we're facing."

"Yes, and these gatekeeping and triage decisions are big ones, because they are crucial for proper diagnosis and treatment initiation," Evelyn emphasized. "However, at the current time, it is quite difficult to know how well the challenge is being met due to the uncertainties regarding what kind of triage process is best for what kinds of problems. We do know that if primary care physicians are responsible for triage, patient care gets sacrificed unless the physicians' education and skills improve. For other kinds of triage, we need comparative studies to assess cost-effectiveness and the impact on informed consent, confidentiality, and other ethical concerns."

"How about including the police, hairdressers, and bartenders as gatekeepers," Adam said—only partly in jest. "Anyway, maybe this is the time for an ethical exhibition game between us," Adam suggested. "How about these scoring guidelines?"

- *Both healthcare and business ethics win* if triage is conducted by those more cost-effective in its process, using a consensus-based definition of "medical necessity" for determining when, who, and what kind of behavioral healthcare is needed.
- *Business ethics win but healthcare ethics lose* if triage is done in unstudied ways designed to control costs, without a concomitant concern for how that affects access and necessary treatment.
- *Healthcare ethics win but business ethics lose* if clinicians insist on triage by particular behavioral healthcare disciplines without concern for cost-effectiveness.

• *Both sides lose* if triage continues in all its unstudied formats and medical necessity is subjectively and secretly defined by each managed care system.

Evelyn agreed to these ethical scoring guidelines. On the way out, Ricky the reviewer caught her and said, "I forgot to bring up in the conference that the prospective patient had complained that she was never provided helpful information about our gatekeeping and triage process and how attention deficit disorder was supposed to be covered, let alone the guarded responses she received from her first contacts."

"Sounds like some informed consent ethical issues," mused Evelyn to Ricky. But there was something more than just what Ricky said that bothered Evelyn. Why had Ricky forgotten to bring up such an important problem? And why did Ricky seem both excited and worried at the same time?

Those questions lead us to the next chapter in the story of The Ethical Way.

COMMENTARY ON CHAPTER FOUR

How does one take care of the employer, take care of the patient, take care of the provider, and take care of oneself (the business)? To answer that, one has to know the historical context of the problem. In the past, when medical costs were rising faster than inflation, behavioral costs were rising four times faster than medical. Attempts at utilization review by medically oriented personnel proved ineffective. Behavioral experts were needed and so carve-out was born. Costs were reduced by making sure that only those who "truly needed" behavioral care got it and the care that was given was "medically necessary" and "appropriate." Medical costs went down and behavioral care became a commodity. Given a set price per member per month, there is a clear push to make sure that the services are the most cost-effective and only delivered to those who truly need them, as well as limited to those covered by the plan the employer bought. Triage, a thoughtful referral to the best place to get the particular help the patient needs, can too easily give way to an approach more reminiscent of a sentry at the gate aggressively guarding the pool of limited resources. So what is our responsibility to each of the stakeholders?

The Patient

Problem: patients have problems that may be the cause of behavioral symptoms (anxiety, depression, sleeplessness, lack of concentration, and so on) that may or may not be linked to true, full-blown behavioral disorders. What the patient wants and needs is help and assurance, not an inquisition. The patient wants triage, true triage. Common triage points prior to direct access to behavioral intake often include EAP, primary care practitioners, and help lines—which are more like telephonic EAP and can direct the patient to elder care services, legal help, financial counseling, human resources help, and so on. Working with those that exist to come to mutual agreement about the responsibilities of each is both helpful to the business and to the patient. But sometimes the patient wants to bypass all of these. Then the managed care must triage genuinely and not just create obstacles. The intake process can begin the evaluation but rarely will allow the time for true triage. Evaluation and diagnostic skills require specific training and so it is that at my organization 99 percent of those who call will get at a minimum a face-to-face evaluation, generally by a social worker who is an expert in evaluation and who, in conjunction with psychiatric consultation and backup, is skilled at making referrals for further medical or psychiatric evaluation and treatment.

At the same time, the efficiency of this process can be enhanced by increasing the skills of the other referral sources with education for primary care practitioners (including screening tools—we have developed telephonic access to the SDDS-PC for patients referred by their primary care physicians), and work with EAP to delineate responsibilities possibly including the development of a telephonic advice line. Finally, the real key to demand management is prevention. Materials such as those developed by the American Institute of Preventative Medicine, the Time Life Series, and so on, as well as HMO or business site education, help the patient to become an even better educated and responsible consumer, thereby increasing the appropriateness of self-referral. Ultimately, however, there is only one rule: when somebody calls in pain and needing help, *always* triage.

The Employer

Problem: to be competitive in the business world I need to have the lowest medical costs. I really don't want high utilization. The key here is *appropriate* utilization, which is best assured by solid and accurate diagnosis and evaluation. Secondarily, the key is to begin a dialogue about the relation of total health costs (which include workers' compensation, disability, decreased productivity, absenteeism, and so on) to direct medical costs. It may be that some employers have been very successful at controlling medical costs (demanding a sentrylike approach to access) but the price has been a greater total health cost. In this case a small increase in direct medical costs might effect a large decrease in indirect medical costs. With increased concerns about return to work, we need prompt evaluation and quick referral to treatment options that help effect the most rapid improvement by the patient. Wait and see is not acceptable.

The Provider

Problem: I think what I do will help this patient. Managed care companies must find true provider partners who are honest about their skills and the potential for improving the patient's symptoms. Outcomes evaluation systems and provider profiling in the context of self-managed networks are key issues in helping determine not only that the issue really is a behavioral illness but also one where there is significant likelihood of making an impact on quality of life, on symptoms, on functioning. Openly shared definitions of medical necessity, level of care guidelines, and practice guidelines are also essential, as well as a commitment to evaluate new treatment approaches and the value they bring.

The Business

If the goal of business truly is to gain and retain new customers, openness about guidelines and processes is essential. All the stakeholders' interests must be attended to. While the media may concentrate on the dyad of provider and patient, the business must incorporate the social responsibility of employers, the community, and the shareholders, as well as the providers and the patients.

Where gatekeeping is concerned, we shouldn't build walls. The days of black-belt managed care should be well and truly over. Our job is to responsibly triage people to the help they need.

DAVID WHITEHOUSE, M.D.
Senior Vice President, Corporate Medical Director
MCC Behavioral Care

CHAPTER FIVE

Informed Consent

—∿∿—

We do have an informed consent policy, don't we?" the businessman, Adam Wilder, asked his co-owner of The Ethical Way, the psychiatrist Evelyn Bloom. "It's a confusing concept to me. Can't patients just trust their clinicians to do right by them? Or should it be a warning label, like on food products? All I've seen as a healthcare recipient was something I had to sign before surgery."

"Yes, of course we have a policy on informed consent," Evelyn replied with some exasperation. "Our basic stance is for information to be shared with patients. That's why I was horrified by this issue of *Time* magazine." She dug a magazine out of her desk. The cover showed a gagged physician and the headline "Special Investigation— What Your Doctor Can't Tell You: An In-Depth Look at Managed Care—And One Woman's Fight to Survive." The article described the experience of one patient and her family with a particular managed care system when she developed symptoms of cancer. The reporter highlighted several aspects of the traditional healthcare ethical and legal principle, informed consent, including:

- The patient's husband reportedly did not pay much attention to the details of his family health plan. He chose the cheapest of three options.

- The husband said he did not get a copy of the full contract until sometime after signing.

- The managed care company had a billboard slogan, "When You've Got Your Health Net, You've Got Everything."

- There were standard operational processes for making referrals, which the patient apparently did not understand and which her oncologist did not follow.

- One physician wondered if patients aren't being told of all the options for treatment, especially those that might be deemed experimental or investigative.

These aspects of the case all brought up questions about how managed care is handling informed consent.

Suddenly more serious, Adam added, "Well, we sure don't need that kind of publicity."

"Unfortunately, we may already be on the way. Remember that woman with attention deficit disorder we were talking about—the one who had trouble with our gatekeeping process? Well, she's starting to complain about some things that have to do with informed consent."

"Such as?" asked Adam.

"Just look at this letter."

Dear The Ethical Way:

After I picked my insurance, I received a copy of your brochure on The Ethical Way. I know I may have a condition for which there is some professional disagreement. All the more reason to have open communication. So how would you explain that:

1. I never received any information about whether adult attention deficit disorder was considered a psychiatric diagnosis in terms of coverage.

2. I wasn't given any information at first about which clinicians were expert in the area, so I found someone on my own, only to be told she wasn't in the network.

3. I asked my doctor if he had any financial incentive on referring me out, but he said he couldn't answer that. I want to know how much of each dollar is spent on patient care, since a survey I read, done by *Bloomberg Personal* magazine, apparently found that the better-rated HMOs spent about 90 cents of every dollar on patient care.

4. I wasn't given clear reasons why neuropsychological testing was not offered to help confirm my diagnosis.

5. I was told that someone deemed insight-oriented therapy for adult ADD as "experimental."

6. You never provided any information on outcomes.

7. I preferred to see a woman clinician, but I was told you don't make referrals on this basis.

I would appreciate an explanation.

Sincerely,
I.C. (See name on envelope.)

P.S. Please keep my name and concerns CONFIDENTIAL.

"Sounds like some significant concerns," Adam replied.

"Yes," Evelyn responded. "Although we have a broad policy on sharing information with patients, it looks like something went awry in its application. Or maybe it was too general, or misunderstood, or even wrong. Perhaps the clinicians she saw didn't inform her as expected. Or the information we previously got from our reviewer, Ricky, was inaccurate."

"Or can the patient be distorting something?" Adam asked.

"Sure," replied Evelyn. "You're getting clinically astute!"

"Thanks, but what do you think we should do?" Adam asked.

"Well, let's go over her points to see what kind of ethics-based response we can make, perhaps in a letter back to her," Evelyn replied. "For instance, give me a minute to check on whether adult attention deficit disorder is a covered diagnosis."

"So what did you find out?" Adam asked.

"I called the benefits officer in the personnel office at the payer. She said they aren't sure either. ADD for children is certainly covered. We discussed how this was becoming a more standardly accepted diagnosis with helpful treatment that would likely improve I.C.'s functioning at work. Then the payer agreed this should be covered and clarified in the next communication about benefits."

"Good, that makes sense," Adam added.

"I.C.'s second point was not receiving enough information about clinical experts for adult ADD," Evelyn continued. "That just doesn't make sense from what Ricky said was done at the case conference."

"Well, maybe for now we can apologize and explain our credentialing process," Adam suggested.

"Good idea. In our credentialing process, we did ask providers about special expertise and we will try over time to verify that their special expertise is really what they say it is."

"We'll really need our outcome project data for that, right?" asked Adam.

"Yes, and that will take a while, but we can tell I.C. that it is in the works," Evelyn replied. "For that third point I.C. makes, I'm not sure why the primary care physician she saw first wouldn't tell her whether he had any potential financial benefit for referring her out. We've never told any clinicians that they couldn't share such information. Either our policy wasn't clear or the physician was just too uncomfortable or unused to discussing such matters."

"Or maybe the physician was following the policies of other managed care companies he deals with," added Adam.

"Agreed," Evelyn replied. "I recently read an editorial in the *American Medical News* that provided a typical contract proviso along the line that the physician should make no communication to enrollees that could undermine the confidence of enrollees in the plan. I.C.'s fourth point also seems like some sort of communication confusion. Why wouldn't one of her clinicians provide clear reasons why neuropsychological testing was not offered? Although helpful in some complex or unusual cases, in my opinion it really doesn't offer much diagnostic help and might use up half of her $1,800 outpatient benefit."

"Right; that seemed true with my boys," Adam added. "Though testing was discussed, the learning disabilities specialist was able to put together all the information to make a diagnosis confidently."

Evelyn continued down the list. "I.C.'s fifth point about why she was told that insight-oriented therapy for ADD was considered experimental is an interesting one. After all, insight-oriented psychotherapy is a time-tested—and partially research-tested—treatment for many psychiatric disorders. But we've also found it not helpful for certain things like bipolar disorders or conditions caused by documentable brain damage. For attention deficit disorder in children, it also hasn't been especially helpful, particularly if the concentration and restlessness isn't controlled first. However, I did just read an article by Carl Sherman that gave a good justification for insight-oriented psychotherapy for adults with attention deficit disorder. The rationale is that insight-oriented therapy would help patients to reconceptualize themselves by exploring how the ADD symptoms led to shame and a negative self-image. Does that sound like an experimental treatment, Adam?"

"No, it doesn't. It seems more like an expected adaptation of a standard treatment. More studies on its effectiveness would be helpful, though."

"I.C.'s sixth point was about not providing information on outcomes," Evelyn continued. "That, too, we are planning, which we can tell her."

"But what about that last point of hers?" Adam asked. "That she wanted to see a woman clinician."

"Yes, I could see the importance of that for some problems, such as remnants of abuse by men, but why for this disorder?" wondered Evelyn.

"Perhaps it's just a basic matter of trust," Adam suggested.

"You really are catching on clinically!" Evelyn replied with a smile of slight embarrassment.

"So let's offer it if she wants it," Adam suggested.

"Agreed," Evelyn replied. "I'll compose a letter per our conversation, which we can both sign."

"Good," Adam replied. "I hope that will be the last we hear of I.C."

"Me, too," said Evelyn. "But I was thinking. Maybe we can learn something from this interaction that can help us to provide better informed consent in the future. Remember when we talked earlier about using an outside ethics consultant to help us look objectively at ethical challenges? This looks like the time to start."

They then contacted Sun-Yu Moon, and after a few days of tough negotiations on the consultation fee, they were ready to continue. They chose Sun-Yu for her Ph.D. in psychology and for her professional reputation as someone with a clear view of cooperative and mutually beneficial outcomes, which might help her to balance the tendency of managed care to focus on competition and profits. They gave her a synopsis of the I.C. case. By then, I.C. had received the letter of explanation. Evelyn had also phoned to talk over the situation, and advised that I.C. seemed to accept their explanation and apology.

"So, Sun-Yu, is there any other way we could or should respond to I.C.?" asked Adam.

"Well, Adam, as the old proverb goes, 'When a man is in great haste he is apt to drink his tea with a fork.'" Adam looked a little displeased and perplexed. "I'd like to give you a quick answer, which I can do, but it may help you to appreciate the complexity of the ethical issues involved, as well as giving you a basis to handle informed consent in the future, for me to give you a little more of the background first. It may seem a little boring, but it will probably be good for you."

"OK, especially if it will help us to handle such issues on our own in the future so we don't have to pay exorbitant consultation fees," replied Adam with a smile. "How about a tea break?"

THE HISTORY OF INFORMED CONSENT IN HEALTHCARE

"The first thing you should know," Sun-Yu began, "is that informed consent is not a traditional healthcare ethical guideline. Nothing about providing patient information or consent is in the Hippocratic Oath. It wasn't even in the AMA Principles of Medical Ethics until 1980. Although perhaps having its roots in European political philosophy, dating back to the Reformation's affirmation of the individual, it was given a boost in modern times with the Nuremberg Code of 1946, following Nazi medical experimentation, and then with political changes in the 1960s in the United States. With the rise of bioethics, patient autonomy and the right to know became a valued counterpart to medical paternalism. In addition, the ethical fiduciary principle of putting the patient first would require not only disclosure about treatment options, but also disclosure about any potential conflict of interest for the clinician.

"The general ethical principle in any form of informed consent is that the clinician will try to choose what seems best for the patient and obtain some sort of implicit or explicit consent to go ahead. However, how much to tell for adequate consent is often unclear, as various aspects of the medical condition may be relevant for the patient to know: diagnosis, choice of treatments, the clinician's expertise in various treatments, the methods that will be used, risks, expected results, and prognosis. How much any given patient will understand about such information will also vary."

Special Aspects of Behavioral Healthcare

"Is there anything different in behavioral healthcare in particular?" asked Adam.

"Ah, yes," replied Sun-Yu. "In the behavioral healthcare field, the concept of informed consent becomes even more complicated. Due to the effects of psychiatric disorders on thinking, emotions, and behavior, the ability of patients to understand the nature of proposed treatments and outcomes may be compromised. Although such an effect may be more obvious when extreme psychosis produces limited reality testing, more subtle effects can ensue from most any disorder."

"Your speaking of psychosis, Sun-Yu," Evelyn added, "reminds me how difficult it is to apply informed consent to schizophrenic patients, who have problems processing information anyway. I can just imagine what it's going to be like when we try to convey managed care information to them. We'll try to describe benefits and the patient will say, 'Whose benefits, yours or mine, is this for a benefit ball or what?' Then try to explain limited numbers of authorized sessions and you may get back, 'You don't like me, do you? Are you going to call the authorities? My old therapist used to see me every week and we'd just talk about what I did every day. I've got insurance, but I can't get anywhere.'"

Sun-Yu laughed and then replied, "It seems like you'll have to gear your information to the patients' capabilities to understand. Anyway, another problem is that providing information to significant others often cannot be done due to patient preference for confidentiality and possible disagreement among significant others.

"The range of helpful treatments is another unique aspect of behavioral healthcare that necessitates extensive disclosure. Much research has indicated that the relationship with the therapist and expectations of improvement are as important—or more so—than the particular type of psychotherapy. Many different kinds of medication can potentially achieve similar results. How to convey such commonalities among treatment options with what may be specifically more indicated for a given patient is a major challenge for informed consent.

"The stigma and myths surrounding mental illness also complicate informed consent. The stigma limits accurate word-of-mouth sharing of information among the public. Antipsychiatry groups may spread erroneous information about certain treatments, especially medications.

"Financial coverage is usually more limited. Unless the patient understands that, developing closeness and trust with a therapist may be shattered if psychotherapy can't proceed for financial reasons.

"The variety of professionals who can provide similar treatments is also different in behavioral healthcare. The public may not understand the differences among psychiatrists, psychologists, therapists, social workers, and psychiatric nurses, even though all of them can provide similar psychotherapy. The public may also be confused as to who can prescribe medication.

"Another unique aspect of behavioral healthcare treatment can be its privacy. Psychotherapy is often conducted with only a therapist and patient involved. There may not even be a secretary around, let alone nurses, other physicians, or other personnel who are more common in other aspects of healthcare to provide information and answer some questions."

"So what's still left in common with general healthcare is the right to be fully informed about treatment options, and the right to get second opinions and refuse treatment unless court ordered." Evelyn commented.

"Correct," replied Sun-Yu, "and legal statutes have supported those ethical principles, at least up to now."

Problems with Informed Consent

"So it seems like with our mental health patients, all we need to be is a little more careful with confidentiality and to be sure the patient is not distorting what is being said." Adam commented.

"Also ethically correct," replied Sun-Yu, "but there is still more to the story about informed consent. Given the newness of informed consent as an ethical healthcare principle, it may not be surprising that questions about the ethical appropriateness of informed consent have arisen. The courts themselves have produced only limited legal guidelines as to how much information is necessary to convey for informed consent. Moreover, the well-known bioethicist Robert Veatch has recently argued that there are multiple problems with the concept of informed consent, including:

"There is no reason to assume that a healthcare clinician who is expert in only one component of well-being should be able to determine what constitutes the good for a patient.

"Even medical well-being may have different—and potentially competing—goods, including preservation of life, cure, reducing suffering, and enhancing health.

"Medical specialists may tend to overvalue their particular field.

"Patients may not want a particular medical good pursued if it comes at the expense of goods in other spheres (including social, financial, religious, occupational, or aesthetic) or if the patient's total well-being may be compromised.

"The good of other parties should also be taken into account.

"Knowing what would seem to be in the best interests of the person does not settle the question of what would be right to do.

"Even if a clinician has good empathy into a patient's values, unconscious factors may influence the clinician's interpretation of scientific data and judgment about what may be best."

These points left the group in deep thought.

The Business Perspective on Informed Consent

Noticing that the effects of the proverb (or of the tea) must be wearing off, Evelyn asked Adam whether the principle of informed consent had relevance in business.

"Yes, but it seems to have a much different meaning. Informed consent in business usually translates to telling the prospective customer whatever is required by law, such as the ingredients in food. Information about a product may intentionally be kept to a minimum so as not to reveal trade secrets to the public or rival businesses. Translating that business ethic to managed care may explain the propensity of many managed care companies to communicate minimally about financial matters, benefit levels, operational processes, and criteria for services. Up until recently, there were virtually no laws that required payers or managed care companies to disclose information on cost control mechanisms to actual or potential beneficiaries."

Evelyn responded, "It seems that such a business orientation runs counter to the developing ethical and legal guidelines for informed consent in healthcare, leading to conflict and confusion."

"Well, I wouldn't completely agree with that statement, Evelyn," Adam replied. "The managed care companies basically want frustrated clinicians to discuss their concerns with plan staff first rather than with patients and the general public. Managed care companies would even say that another reason for controlling information would coincide with the healthcare ethic of putting the patient's interests first, which is for clinicians to discuss with the managed care company what might be the best treatment possible under the circumstances for the patient before making a recommendation to the patient."

"So how should we resolve these differing ethical perspectives in behavioral managed care operation, Sun-Yu?" Evelyn asked.

"Very carefully," replied Sun-Yu. "As the old Chinese proverb goes, 'measure your feet before you buy shoes.' The key difference with managed care is that not only does informed consent involve what is communicated between clinician and patient, but what is communicated across the whole system. Since managed care is usually associated with specific benefit limitations or approval processes for treatment, proper informed consent would include communication to the patient about those influences on treatment."

THE EFFECTS OF MANAGED CARE

"And how well has managed care been doing in general with informed consent?" asked Evelyn.

"Not too well, it seems," replied Sun-Yu. "While there do not seem to be any direct comparative studies of informed consent in managed care versus traditional healthcare, Heather Fields and others recently reported on certain patterns that seem to be emerging, including:

"Many patients seem unaware of the nature, rules, regulations, and varieties of managed care.

"Many patients seem unaware of how a gatekeeping process may work.

"The public and patients have not participated in the dialogue about the use of utilization review.

"Employers vary in how much they have checked out the characteristics of plans offered for their employees.

"The public generally only knows their monthly premiums, but not necessarily the financial parameters of their mental health benefits.

"Written or verbal gag clauses prohibit many clinicians from discussing certain matters with patients, including the range of possible treatments, referral sources, bonus arrangements, or any criticism of the managed care company."

Guidelines for Clinicians

"That so-called gag clause has been really difficult for clinicians," Evelyn added. "Many healthcare professional associations are recommending that clinicians must ethically ignore such prohibitions if they feel they are counter to the patient's best interest. However, if you go against it, the managed care company may stop referrals. And I can hardly believe this extension of the gag clause I heard about in Milwaukee, where both an employee and a referral source were threatened with job loss and patient loss if they continued to remain on the editorial board of the *Canary,* a local newsletter with commentary— from all perspectives—on managed care and psychotherapy. If clinicians decide to comply with the gag clauses, they lose their right of free speech and run the risk of being viewed as professionally unethical and at legal risk for malpractice."

"So what would you suggest we tell our clinicians about informed consent, Sun-Yu?" demanded Adam.

"Ah, Adam, ever wanting to get down to the practical and the nittygritty," replied Sun-Yu. "However, as another old proverb says, 'A hundred lifetimes may not be enough to rectify the mistake made in one morning.' But here is what I would suggest you consider telling your clinicians, perhaps in a more specific policy and procedure format than you currently have:

"*Policy:* Inform patients on the first visit of the nature of their insurance benefits as they might influence therapeutic decisions, confidentiality, and patient choice. However, do so in an accurate, emotionally neutral manner so as not to jeopardize the alliance among the managed care company, provider, and patient.

"*Procedure:* For example, treatment options for a patient with symptoms of a posttraumatic stress disorder could range from techniques to reduce the symptoms to more definitive psychotherapy to process earlier childhood sexual abuse. So the patient could be told:

Ms. Smith, you have what we call a posttraumatic stress disorder. Your poor sleep, memory lapses, and depression likely are coming from a new relationship that is reminding you of the earlier trauma you mentioned. There are several treatment options to consider. Medication can reduce the intensity of the symptoms and some biweekly cognitive therapy can help you to manage your reactions. That kind of treatment would likely fit under your insurance benefits, though I still would need to receive authorization for payment from the managed care company. If for some reason we don't receive authorization, I would appeal it and you could also contact the reviewer or your employer. There is also more extensive treatment available that might help you get over the original trauma and help you to be much less vulnerable in the future. That would be more intensive weekly or twice-weekly insight-oriented psychotherapy. You should also know that there is still a lot of uncertainty and even controversy as to the accuracy of early memories and the best treatment for the aftermath of childhood trauma. If you desired the more intensive therapy, I'm not sure if your plan has the best specialists in this area, so you might have to pay out-of-pocket or petition your plan.

"*Policy:* After discussing treatment options, the clinician should discuss confidentiality.

"*Procedure:* Let the patient know who the clinician may need to share information with, such as:

General behavioral healthcare ethical and legal guidelines require that certain things cannot be held in confidence. These things cover danger to self or others, including suicide risk, homicide risk, suspected child or elder abuse, and sometimes inability to care for oneself. In addition, your managed care plan requires that I share some information with a plan reviewer in order to choose the most cost-effective treatment for you. However, to do so, I may have to share some intimate information, including about your current sex life and the possible perpetrators of your childhood sexual abuse. If I have to do so, is that all right with you?

"*Policy:* The patient should not be coerced, directly or indirectly, into any particular treatment, but rather given any information to make an informed choice.

"*Procedure:* Let the patient make the final choice with all pertinent information:

So, Ms. Smith, the final choice is yours. Before you make the choice, you should know that your managed care plan can provide bonuses to clinicians who provide the most cost-effective treatment, including me. I myself do not have any special expertise in the treatment of post-traumatic stress disorder. I do know some male and female clinicians who specialize in this area if you want to see someone else. The most important consideration is that we select the treatment that best suits your needs at this time.

"*Policy:* To document such discussions, the clinician may want to complete some general written informed consent form with the patient. Your procedure should leave room for patient individuality.

"Procedure: "In part because there are so many ways to write an informed consent form—"

"Yes, of course," Evelyn broke in. "With behavioral healthcare patients, the amount and timing of information presented needs to be considered in view of the patient's mental problems:

"Patients with prior trauma shouldn't be assaulted with unwanted information and should not feel violated or coerced.

"Paranoid patients need utmost openness.

"Anxious patients may require information in small, manageable quantities.

"Schizophrenic patients may require clear, repetitive information.

"Patients with limited mental functioning may need information shared with significant others."

"That sounds ethically correct," answered Sun-Yu. "That's another reason to have a general informed consent form that will be supplemental to verbal consent according to patients' needs."

"Those policies and procedures look helpful for our clinicians," Evelyn continued after lunch. I think we can go ahead and devise a more specific informed consent agreement to document that the clinician has discussed insurance benefits, treatment options, confidentiality, patient choice, and financial influences."

Other Solutions

"What else do you think we should do to improve our approach to informed consent?" asked Evelyn.

Sun-Yu further discussed the ideas of Robert Veatch, who argues that even at its best, informed consent has limited ethical benefits for patients. He maintains that unless there is a deeper sharing of values among clinicians, patients, and their insurance coverage, any routine recommendation of treatment may not be able to take the patient's best interest into enough account. Such limitations can be most obvious in cross-cultural interactions. For example, recommending individual psychotherapy to a patient coming from a traditional Asian culture may run counter to that individual's cultural values of putting family and cultural harmony before individual needs. "So one other solution for The Ethical Way is to have enough behavioral healthcare plan choices to reflect different value frameworks. For instance, you might develop in your network a feminist orientation, holistic health treatment, a particular religious orientation, or particular cultural expertise. Veatch even suggests that informed consent may not go far enough, and that we need a new healthcare ethical principle with a more radical notion of active patient participation in choosing among plausible alternatives."

Sun-Yu also thought that some of the basic informed consent ethical problems needed legislation, which was beyond the influence of Adam and Evelyn. She had read that Massachusetts recently enacted legislation barring the so-called gag clauses from contracts. In many states, medical societies and hospital associations are pressing for legislation that will produce regulations that managed care organizations outline the utilization review criteria and procedures that are used to make funding authorization decisions.

Sun-Yu realized that I.C., the patient who had provoked the ethics consultation, was unusual. Most patients will not realize what they're missing or protest if something seems wrong. There probably need to be some independent watchdog organizations to help them know they need to be aware that shopping for the best health plan or behavioral health plan is not the same as shopping for the best deal on a car between different dealerships. The cheapest plan may not be the best or most cost-effective. She suggested that The Ethical Way consider developing and publicizing a managed care advisory service—akin to a personal financial advisor—to help patients understand their benefits, amount of coverage, and options.

Much more careful thought and discussion would be needed. She thought of another old proverb: "Let your ideas be round but your conduct square."

BUSINESS VERSUS BEHAVIORAL
HEALTHCARE ETHICS SCORECARD

As the ethics consultation on informed consent broke up, Evelyn and Adam felt that both The Ethical Way and managed behavioral healthcare in general had a formidable challenge to resolve the various business and healthcare ethical issues on informed consent. The goals include making sure that patients are as informed as they want and need to be, clinicians can comfortably follow the ethical guidelines of their profession, and healthcare systems can be successful in a business sense to produce cost-effective treatment. Adam and Evelyn agreed to a competition that would be scored as follows:

- *Both healthcare and business ethics win* if informed consent guidelines can be developed that simultaneously incorporate the new informational complexities of managed care, protect necessary proprietary interests, support clinicians' ethical and legal responsibilities to their patients, and satisfy the consumer's need to know relevant information.

- *Business ethics win but healthcare ethics lose* if managed care companies are allowed to keep information hidden that will hamper a therapeutic alliance and appropriate treatment.

- *Healthcare ethics win but business ethics lose* if every endeavor is made to obtain any possible relevant information for the consumer, but the process is so time-consuming and comprehensive that it is no longer cost-effective.

- *Both sides lose* if the current confusion and controversy about informed consent is allowed to continue and the *Time* magazine cover story Evelyn showed Adam doesn't become obsolete.

As they bid good-bye that late Friday afternoon, they thanked Sun-Yu, mentioning that they were sure she would be needed again. Before the door closed, they were stopped by an out-of-breath staff member, who quickly blurted out, "It looks like we've got another problem with that patient, I.C. It seems like somehow information on her condition got to her office and she's threatening to sue us for breach of confidentiality." Somehow Evelyn wasn't completely surprised. She didn't think it was I.C.'s clinician who could have breached confidentiality. That clinician had a reputation for watching confidentiality closely, and in fact had for a long time protested having to tell a utilization reviewer any personal information about a patient. But she wondered about that utilization reviewer, Ricky. Her mind drifted back to the end of the administrative case conference on gatekeeping and the discrepancy about who I.C. saw.

COMMENTARIES ON CHAPTER FIVE

The principle of informed consent has roots in law, ethics, and social policy. It is not a principle that comes naturally to many healthcare professionals—in fact, it may collide with professional training that emphasizes that clinicians must determine and act on what is in the best interests of their patients and clients. Designed to assure that patients can exercise autonomy in decision making to the maximum degree possible, it is sometimes viewed as a nuisance, a matter of persuading a patient to sign an informed consent form so that treatment may proceed. The law's insistence that any consequential risk be disclosed may be viewed by some as countertherapeutic if concern regarding risk causes a patient to decline treatment.

Yet informed consent is not simply or primarily about getting a form signed, nor is it intended to further conflict between therapist and client. Rather, as Jay Katz observes in his classic work *The Silent World of Doctor and Patient,* the principle of informed consent should strengthen the therapeutic relationship by causing the parties to that relationship to spend time discussing the views of both clinician and client as to what each considers in the best interests of the client. As Katz points out, both parties relate to each other as equals and as unequals. Healthcare professionals presumably know more about illness and disease while patients know more about their individual needs (which often go beyond symptom reduction). Only open discussion can enable both parties to bring their strengths and weaknesses to decision making regarding treatment—only through such discussion can the trust that must be the basis for good clinical relationships be developed.

At the same time, giving life to informed consent has become more complicated in a managed care environment. Cost has become a much more explicit issue, not only in discussions of health and behavioral healthcare policy generally, but in the setting of the individual treatment relationship. In addition, more behavioral healthcare professionals work for an employer or under contract to a purchaser or payer; these oblig-ations may create economic conflict with the ethical responsibility to act in the best interests of the client. These potential conflicts have given rise to the idea of "economic informed consent," which in prac-tice means assuring that the client understands the economic con-straints on the provision of certain types of treatment.

As the chapter points out, gag rules often have prohibited behav-ioral healthcare professionals from telling clients about contractual lim-itations on treatment. However, such rules—already under challenge because of the ethically untenable position in which they place health-care practitioners—inevitably will give way to legal challenge in the courts and legislatures. As gag rules disappear, and as the imperative to provide clients with all information pertinent to their treatment is extended to economic concerns, clinicians will have to decide how such information is to be made available. The author provides a useful example of how such a conversation might occur in practice. However, the author may underestimate the impact on patients of being told that some potentially helpful treatments are simply unavailable because they are not covered in the plan. For example, most individuals probably do not know that many hospitals have two formularies in practice, one for those with insurance and one for those without. "Economic informed consent" would suggest that this type of information would have to be disclosed to an indigent patient. Will this disclosure create its own set of clinical issues and if so how will those be addressed?

Finally, the author's emphasis on recognizing different values based on culture, gender, and race is critical if informed consent is to become in practice what it is in theory. In 1982, a presidential commission issued a report on the ethical and legal implications of informed con-sent in the patient-practitioner relationship, concluding that informed consent worked best when the socioeconomic status of the healthcare provider and patient were most closely related. On the other hand, poverty and race affected the amount and type of information pro-vided to patients.

Since that time, we have learned much about the differences gen-der makes in treatment in conditions as diverse as cardiac disease and mental illness. We have also learned from the emerging focus on out-comes and on consumerism that the preferences of clients (and their families) may be quite different from practitioner definition of client best interest. This suggests that as informed consent evolves, Jay Katz's view that we must recognize both what is common and not common between client and therapist assumes even greater importance. Without that recognition, and the conversations that must occur to achieve it, informed consent may continue to be viewed as simply a nuisance, rather than as a principle that can foster and reinforce the therapeutic relationship.

JOHN PETRILA, J.D.
Chair, Department of Mental Health Law and Policy
University of South Florida

The largest single issue—often missed in discussions of informed consent—is that informed consent is an ongoing process rather than a one-time activity. That is, issues of informed consent must be addressed repeatedly throughout the entire time that the consumer is receiving services.

There are two reasons why informed consent needs to be a process. First of all, in the case of psychiatric disorders, there are often barriers to the consumer clearly processing information when it is presented. However, it is important also to note that even in nonpsychiatric issues, informed consent needs to be an ongoing process. For example, if a physician tells a patient that the diagnosis involves a serious and possibly fatal illness, this would be so anxiety provoking that the patient likely would not fully understand other information presented at the same time. Therefore, whether regarding psychiatric disorders or otherwise, it is important that consumers have repeated opportunities to increase their depth and accuracy of understanding of the information relevant to the services being rendered.

The other reason that informed consent needs to be a process is that as the treatment progresses, the original course and type of treatment may be modified and it is important to keep the consumer adequately informed.

ALAN L. ZIGLIN, Ph.D.
Executive Director
Northwest Georgia Regional Mental Health,
Mental Retardation, and Substance Abuse Board

CHAPTER SIX

Confidentiality

—《》— **M**y God!" Evelyn Bloom, M.D., co-owner of The Ethical Way, said to her partner, businessman Adam Wilder, "We seem to be getting one ethical problem after another."

"Yes, even with all our preparation," Adam sighed. "And I thought we were done with I.C. after processing the gatekeeping and informed consent ethical problems involving her."

"I've got a hunch who leaked the information on I.C. to her workplace," Evelyn mused. "But first, let me call her to apologize again and tell her we'll investigate and try to help right away."

"And I'll call our lawyer to see if there's anything we should or shouldn't do," Adam added. "So don't say too much to I.C."

"I won't," Evelyn replied. "We seemed to hit it off nicely when I called her before, so I'll try to reestablish some connection so she'll feel we're working on this together. Let's meet again in an hour. Hopefully, we can make these connections even though it's late Friday afternoon. I'm familiar with patient care crises on Friday afternoons; I didn't know administrative ones happen then, too."

"Yes, we administrators don't always get to leave early on Friday to play golf," Adam retorted.

Later, they met again and Adam said that the lawyer felt that they didn't have to do anything yet on the legal side, but that they should try to flesh out the information from I.C. and investigate any suspicions that they had about what happened.

"Sounds fine," said Evelyn. "My call to I.C. has already paid dividends. I called her to apologize again, which she was reluctant to accept, but she was willing to go on talking."

It turned out that the immediate aftermath of the leak had not been too bad. "In fact, the people she works with were curious about what attention deficit disorder meant for adults, anyway, as they were more knowledgeable about its manifestation in children. 'At least they realized I wasn't crazy,' she told me. So I.C. talked more to the director of personnel and her boss to explain some of how she thought ADD was affecting her. Since they valued her, and could see where treatment could improve her functioning, they wanted her to get any help possible. Of course, I offered follow-up education."

"Great," said a relieved Adam. "So it sounds like we're not going to get sued."

"It doesn't seem so," Evelyn responded. "Unless something else goes wrong ethically with I.C."

"With all this attention, discussion, and learning we're doing, I should hope not," Adam commented. "Now, did you get any leads that can help us to figure out how the confidentiality was breached?"

"I did ask I.C. if she had any suspicions of how the information had gotten out. She said she asked who told the company about her problem. The director of personnel said it was some nurse from The Ethical Way. That did get I.C. thinking, and she told me that not long ago she had gotten involved in a triangular relationship and the other woman had threatened revenge. She said she knew that the other woman worked in managed care as a nurse."

For Evelyn, the puzzle was coming together. Ricky, one of their utilization reviewers, was also a nurse and of the same age range as I.C. Not only do utilization reviewers have a lot of access to patient information, but Ricky left out some important information in her presentation of I.C.'s case, then had a strong, ambivalent reaction when the breach of confidentiality was found.

She told Adam and Adam quickly said, "OK, that's enough for me. I'm going to go see Ricky and fire her."

"Wouldn't that be legally risky?" asked Evelyn. "And intimidating. Besides, we're not sure yet. Let me talk to her. We're both women and also have a common professional medical bond."

Evelyn called Ricky to set up an emergency meeting. At the meeting, Evelyn wondered about Ricky's responses to I.C. She also asked Ricky who might have leaked confidential information to I.C.'s workplace. Ricky became more anxious and vague with her responses. When Evelyn mentioned that it seemed to be a nurse whom I.C. knew, Ricky broke down and admitted her unethical behavior. "Even though I'm not functioning as a clinician, I knew it was wrong for a utilization reviewer to share any information that the patient didn't approve. But once I heard a lot of information about the patient and her history, even though our coding protected her name, I knew it was I.C. And I was so angry at her, this was my way to get back. I'm sorry, I know I'll never do this again. I'm willing to resign."

"Thanks for clarifying this problem for us," Evelyn responded, "and we'll accept your resignation. Tell me, if you will, how you contacted her employer so we can undo some of the damage."

"OK. I called the benefits office under the guise of finding out if this was an excluded diagnosis for her insurance company, and I just happened to let slip I.C.'s name in connection with that," Ricky answered.

Ricky did resign, and Evelyn suggested she obtain some psychotherapy, then called I.C. and said that they had found the culprit, who was no longer with The Ethical Way. I.C. asked who it was, and after slight hesitation, Evelyn named Ricky. I.C. was surprised, but satisfied. Evelyn then asked I.C. if there were any recommendations I.C. had for them to avoid such problems in the future. I.C. thought for a while, then said, "Actually, something simple would have worked for me, I think. If I had known that Ricky was to review my case, I could have told my therapist there would be an ethical conflict of interest and you could have assigned someone else. So if you don't keep the names of reviewers confidential, that should help."

Evelyn later met with Adam to update him.

"You did great," Adam commented.

"Thanks, it looks like the fire is out, at least for now. But I sense we should bring back Sun-Yu to process this and learn even more about confidentiality challenges in managed care to see what changes we should make. We barely touched on them when we discussed confidentiality as part of informed consent."

"Yes, I agree. I know this is going to cost us more money and I can't stand those allegedly old proverbs, but we'd better bring her back."

After being briefed on I.C. again, Sun-Yu began with yet another old saying, "Coarse people leave their door open by an inch, lazy people leave it open by three inches, but only complete idiots leave it wide open."

"Now I don't mean you've been complete idiots about confidentiality. No, rather it is because privacy can be so important to your patients that opening doors to personal information can be very perilous. Here, too, history is important to understand. Is it all right with you, Adam, to cover some of that history?"

"Yes, if that will help with all the ethical problems we're having."

"And I promise no more proverbs on this subject. I think you got the message. In contrast to informed consent, confidentiality has been a major healthcare guideline since at least the Hippocratic Oath, which says, 'Whatever things I see or hear concerning the life of man, in any attendance on the sick or even apart therefrom, which ought not to be voiced about, I will keep silent thereon . . . '"

"Yes, even I have heard of the Hippocratic Oath," interrupted Adam. "But there seems to be a key phrase here, 'which ought not to be voiced about,' which seems to indicate that confidentiality wasn't meant to be absolute."

"Ethically correct," acknowledged Sun-Yu. "And that is precisely why so many ethical issues have arisen around confidentiality. Even legally, the response to confidentiality in healthcare has been ambiguous. Although as of 1996, thirty-four states have laws on medical record confidentiality, most of these laws are so limited that they offer little protection. So it will be up to us to try to determine what information 'ought not to be voiced about' in The Ethical Way."

CONFIDENTIALITY STANDARDS

"Let's examine in more detail how confidentiality has been viewed in behavioral healthcare before the rise of managed care," continued Sun-Yu after a break. "Most authorities, including Thomas Gutheil, Robert Goldstein, and Christopher Bolas, emphasize that confidentiality may be even more crucial in behavioral healthcare than the rest of healthcare. Though never studied in a double-blind research way, it is assumed that confidentiality helps any patient to reveal problems or let his or her body be examined. In behavioral healthcare, given the personal nature of problems along with the remaining stigma of mental health problems, confidentiality is assumed to be even more critical in order to allow patients to reveal private thoughts and emotions that will help ensure accurate diagnosis and treatment. Clinicians are not even supposed to discuss patients with their spouses. If such confidential information would be revealed to the wrong parties, damaging effects such as shame, stigma, and even insurance or job loss could ensue."

"Well, we've sure seen that with our patient I.C.," added Adam. "She seemed ashamed at her behavioral problems being made public and thought her job was in jeopardy."

"Yes, and by the way, I just met with people at her job to let them know more about ADD and that it's not a condition for which they should penalize an employee," Evelyn added. "They now seem to realize that although attention deficit disorder does limit some of her capabilities, she's developed extraordinary compensatory mechanisms, and treatment should help her to function even better.

"You know, over the years some patients of mine have been willing to self-pay, at great personal expense, so as to avoid any information going to an insurance company, and have asked that my notes be kept in a special place."

"Did you agree to keep notes in a special place?" asked Sun-Yu.

"With much reservation, yes. I thought it was more important to get them into treatment than to comply with our standard clinical record-keeping system. Maybe I should have talked to you then."

"Perhaps. What if you were unavailable and a future clinician needed your records?" asked Sun-Yu. "But I'm sure many clinicians would agree with you. In psychoanalysis, complete confidentiality, including minimal note taking, has been assumed to be crucial for the process to even take place, so as to remove any outside influence on the 'blank screen' of the analysis."

"Well, that's very interesting from a theoretical framework, and maybe helpful for the patient," Adam interjected. "On the other hand, keeping information confidential may cause other kinds of problems, particularly for society as a whole. Not allowing enough information to go out leaves third-party payers unsure of what they are paying for."

"Yes, I can appreciate that business perspective," replied Evelyn. "Moreover, limited written information will not allow certain kinds of research projects and measurement of quality of care to take place. Such research would be especially compromised by the prior tendency of many clinicians to underdiagnose on an insurance form in order to minimize the seriousness of the disorder, an ethical issue of honesty in itself."

"Nothing you've ever been guilty of, I'm sure," Sun-Yu said with a smile.

"Well, perhaps once or twice, at least," admitted Evelyn a bit sheepishly. "In the days prior to managed care, when a patient asked me to be careful about what I put on a reimbursement insurance form because it might somehow get back to work or make it difficult to obtain life insurance, it was hard not to stretch the truth for the patient's good."

MEETING CONFIDENTIALITY STANDARDS

"Given the special concerns in the mental health field for confidentiality, yet with the tendency of all of us to fall short of our ideals, how well has confidentiality been handled?" Sun-Yu asked, and proceeded to begin to answer herself.

"If we look over the twenty or thirty years before managed care, it appears that while one can assume appropriate handling of confidentiality by most clinicians and institutions, there have been breaches of confidentiality for various reasons. What seemed to be the most innocuous breach, just opening the proverbial confidentiality door a fraction of an inch, began with increasing third-party coverage of psychiatric treatment in the 1960s and 1970s. To receive payment for psychotherapy or hospitalization, all a clinician had to do was fill out a simple insurance form by stating a diagnosis, a treatment plan, and a brief note on progress. But such information was not necessarily processed with patients before being sent out. In addition, on occasion patients would find out even this minimal information had leaked out, compromising trust in the clinician. And when patients requested letters in the 1960s for abortion or the draft boards, Eric Plant reported that the same psychotherapists who advocated for absolute confidentiality would often comply and write letters on their patients' behalf."

"Interesting," Adam responded. "Maybe the public pushed the door open to that full inch. Self-disclosure was all the rage then, which eventually extended to patients, now drastically escalated on the media, especially talk shows. I wouldn't even be surprised to see our patient I.C. on *Oprah* with a panel of other adult victims of attention deficit disorders, showing old report cards and demanding full rights to reeducation."

Sun-Yu laughed and replied, "Just for ethical clarification, here we have the loosening of patient privilege to release information, the counterpart of the clinician's guideline on confidentiality."

"Yes, and Adam is right about societal influences on patient confidentiality," Evelyn continued. "As time went on, other compromises of confidentiality developed. The needs of society to know information gained ground when threats to society were deemed enough for the clinician to break confidentiality. So we had the Tarasoff decision in California setting a precedent for warning identified possible victims of violence from psychiatric patients, and we had laws on reporting child or elder abuse—all told, the duty of the mental health clinician to protect others has been receiving more and more legal and ethical attention. Coincidentally or not, the tradition of camouflaging patient identity in writing up cases seemed to loosen, to include the ethically controversial after-death release of tapes of the treatment of the well-known poet Anne Sexton for the biography by Middlebrook."

"Yes, I think that Sexton case was a mistake," replied Sun-Yu. "After death, a patient may need even more confidentiality protection, and I don't see how the release of the treatment tapes was in society's best needs."

"Other than perhaps to make the public more aware of confidentiality issues," Adam added. "And it certainly was an interesting book."

"Back to our review," Sun-Yu admonished, for the first time showing a little impatience herself. "In the midst of these concerns about confidentiality, some research was conducted to see how well mental health clinicians were actually doing in protecting confidentiality. A Canadian study in 1980 found numerous releases of confidential personal information to third parties that were not authorized by patients. As part of that study, insurance companies using private investigators were able to obtain confidential medical and psychiatric information in over 75 percent of the patient-related contacts they made at hospitals or medical offices, usually due to carelessness or an absence of safeguards. That the medical facility even acknowledged that an individual was a patient was breaking ethical standards of confidentiality that are so important in behavioral healthcare.

"In a related experiment, a law student was able to obtain records from psychiatric facilities on two patients without their knowledge or consent. And in 1987, when Pope studied more than five hundred U.S. psychologists, well over half admitted that they had inadvertently breached a patient's confidentiality. Over 75 percent admitted that they had discussed patients with friends, and 8 percent of those admitted naming the patient. The study did not even include such routine breaches of confidentiality as talking about patients in public areas such as elevators, or discussing patients with colleagues not connected to the case."

"That sure fits my experience as a layman," Adam added. "Maybe it's because I haven't been in the health field, but I often hear comments about mental patients in public places. Juicy stuff sometimes, but embarrassing. How have the behavioral healthcare associations responded to all of this?"

Sun-Yu continued, "The responses of professional associations to these ethical quandaries or breaches have varied. As more information was demanded and relayed to others, most professional groups were—perhaps unfortunately—relatively silent. While patient privilege to approve or disapprove release of information is some kind of safeguard, it is limited by what patients may understand about what is to be released, as well as by unconscious influences within patients on whether they will comply or not."

THE INFLUENCE OF MANAGED CARE

"So if this all wasn't complicated enough, then we add the effects of managed care systems," Adam commented.

"Yes," Sun-Yu agreed. "Managed care companies generally ask for much more information than third parties have traditionally requested from clinicians. The ethical explanations given for such requests generally have fallen into two categories. One is based on the known history of some clinicians to distort information on forms, which we already discussed. Then managed care companies began to discover that some clinicians charged for sessions not provided or approved. A more general reason applicable to all clinicians is to make sure that the intended treatment meets criteria of medical necessity as designated in the third-party benefits. In addition to treatment plans, managed care companies will often ask for copies of any notes kept on patients; they sometimes do on-site reviews of charts in hospitals, and on occasion they even talk directly to the patient to try to verify information."

"Actually call a patient, you said?" asked Adam in some disbelief.

"Yes, it does sound a little unusual," Evelyn agreed. "But I approved that just the other day for one of our utilization reviewers. Not Ricky! There was a patient of ours who had gone to the emergency room wanting admission to the hospital. The patient said she was suicidal and had used all her money on cocaine. The emergency room psychiatrist believed her. There was no psychosis. Her family hadn't been contacted for any verification. Fortunately, the reviewer recognized the patient's name and that she had been to other emergency rooms in the past with similar claims. One of our clinicians had warned the on-call reviewer that this could happen. Once the reviewer got on the phone with the patient, after some resistance from the emergency room, the patient admitted that she mainly wanted to get off the street and away from her responsibilities. There was nothing new that would verify a higher suicide risk. When we offered her and the emergency room psychiatrist an immediate follow-up at our clinic, they agreed.

Another example is receiving a treatment plan from a network psychiatrist where the diagnosis was a psychotic depression but the patient was not on an antipsychotic. The patient was asked to come in to see one of our mental health gatekeepers to review the treatment. There it became clear that the psychiatrist was making the diagnosis of depression seem worse in order to obtain more authorized sessions for psychotherapy as the primary treatment. I guess here we have the opposite of the prior tendencies of clinicians to underdiagnose on insurance forms. Too bad the psychiatrist didn't realize we weren't one of the companies that refuses to allow psychiatrists to do psychotherapy."

"It seems that having a reviewer talk to the patient can be helpful, but it pushes the door to confidentiality even further," Adam responded. "But it's not as the proverb says, Sun-Yu. Making the call is the opposite of laziness."

RECORD KEEPING

"That is your interpretation, Adam," replied Sun-Yu. "But to continue. To comply with the request of managed care companies to obtain more information—should they choose to comply—clinicians have had to change how they process and record information. One change is what is conveyed in note taking, whether written or electronic."

"Yes, but before you go on to what is put into notes, what do you think about clinicians who do their notes with patients present, not only to be open with patients, but perhaps to add that to their billable time?"

"Very clever, I think," said Sun-Yu, "but perhaps also ethical, as long as the patient doesn't mind, if you want to consider that any time devoted to the care of the patient, whether face-to-face or not, could be justified as reimbursable." After Evelyn and Adam nodded in agreement,

Sun-Yu went on. "Clinicians have had to learn to adapt notes to reflect medical necessity, but spell out the information in terms that even a clerk—who may indeed review the material—would understand."

At the mention of electronic note taking, Adam brightened considerably, fondly remembering his software days. "We want our clinicians to become more familiar with electronic data processing, don't we, Evelyn? Managed care companies are trying to shift in that direction due to estimated cost savings of $90 billion a year. Besides cost savings, Nancy Tracy and Cheryl Kesser-Hoffman have described ways that electronic records can enhance quality of care in several ways:

"One: they increase access to patient care information.

"Two: they provide better information integration over time and across settings.

"Three: they provide information more quickly.

"Four: they provide precision support data for clinicians.

"Five: they reduce redundancy of testing by making results more easily available.

"Six: they let clinicians spend less time hunting for important information on patient care."

"Nevertheless, for all the advantages of electronic note taking," Evelyn cautioned, "clinicians who hospitalize patients also have to be aware that the entire record could be put on-line without the clinician or patient being told. Even speculative information can leak out. Moreover, whenever utilization review is performed, clinicians have to expect to be asked much more detailed information about a patient's history, sometimes including personal sexual histories."

CONFIDENTIALITY CONCERNS

"You both have good points," Sun-Yu continued. "While managed care companies claim that such alterations of confidentiality meet important healthcare ethical standards due to improved monitoring and appropriate treatment, as well as business ethics due to cost savings, others are not so sure that these changes do not come at higher ethical costs."

"Precisely," agreed Evelyn. "Let me share a letter about confidentiality I received from one of our own valuable network clinicians, the psychologist Russ Hagen. Although unsolicited, his comments aren't surprising; we have emphasized openness in our staff and network." Adam and Sun-Yu bent to read the letter together. It said:

Dear Evelyn and Adam:

I welcome the opportunity you've provided for clinicians to share their concerns. While I agree that more sharing of information may be needed to improve patient care, long the goal of traditional case conferences, routine sharing of confidential information in a system brings up some new concerns for me. Among the concerns are the following:

1. *Use of patient information other than for patient care.* One example was reported in Maryland, where Medicaid clerks tapped into computers to obtain and sell the information to HMO recruiters, who then visited the patients to make sales pitches about joining their healthcare system.

2. *Lack of confidentiality safeguards.* In the past, psychiatric records generally seemed to be safe, and even when available may have been illegible. Now it is often unknown what happens to detailed written or electronic information once it is released by the clinician. Information can be misused by anybody, including primary care physicians.

3. *Information availability to nonclinicians.* Reviewers who have no direct contact or clinical relationship with a patient, and who also may not be clinicians themselves, may not be familiar with—or bound to—any healthcare ethics about confidentiality.

4. *Because managed care organizations are businesses, other professional standards and state medical laws may not apply.* Even the National Committee for Quality Assurance, which accredits managed care organizations, so far only assesses confidentiality to the extent that the managed care organization complies with its own standards.

5. *There are no standards for the handling, storage, and destruction of medical records obtained by managed care organizations.* Once they've got the records, anything can happen!

6. *I've read that on the average, seventeen people may see a patient's record in a managed care company.* Isn't that way too many?

Sincerely,
Russ

"Those points are well-taken," replied Adam. "Overall, the key ethical question with all of these concerns is whether and how much patient harm may come from the changes instituted by managed care, and whether the benefits outweigh the risks and problems. So far, it appears to me that the harm is mainly anecdotal and difficult to put into some broader context. Although confidentiality has been a long-standing ethical principle in healthcare, it is apparent that the door to confidentiality always has a tendency to swing open to one degree or another."

SOME SOLUTIONS

"Are we finally ready to adjust our guidelines for confidentiality?" Adam continued. "Or, as some would say, how do we make sure the door to information only opens when it ethically should? And if I put on my consumer hat, isn't the record mine anyway, to do with as I want?"

"Yes, it is yours, Adam, but it's not as simple as that." Evelyn answered. "We already discussed that clinicians may keep important information out of the chart—information that could still get released. And I believe that in the behavioral healthcare arena a clinician has the right not to give records to a patient if the clinician believes that to do so would be harmful to the patient."

"Good. Now I think we've covered all the essential background information," Sun-Yu confirmed. "And although bioethicists usually try to see all sides of ethical issues, this much is very clear to me. Managed care companies must accept the burden of proof that comes with altering such a time-tested, tried-and-true ethical guideline as confidentiality. It is up to managed care companies like yours to prove that their new policies about confidentiality are not unduly harming patients and not unduly compromising traditional healthcare ethics. Although I'm usually not so assertive, I'll repeat myself here. The burden of proof is on managed care companies to be sure that alterations in handling confidentiality—or any time-tested ethical healthcare guideline, for that matter—do not cause more harm than good to patients."

"How do you think we can show that?" asked Evelyn.

"Well, one method of showing that proof is to conduct studies on the effects of looser confidentiality," Sun-Yu suggested. "Such studies could compare groups of patients who would be protected by traditional standards versus newer standards. Patients could be asked directly about any known adverse effects as part of patient satisfaction surveys."

"Agreed," replied Evelyn, "but that's difficult and time-consuming. In addition, isn't it more important for us to educate, monitor, and respond to employees about the importance of confidentiality? This would be especially important for nonclinical employees who are not subject to professional ethical codes as I am. Along this line, developing employees who are content, well-trained, and educated about the adverse consequences of breaking patients' confidentiality needs should help to avoid misuse of personal information. Thinking back to I.C., we can try to improve our character screening of employees, but that's quite difficult due to legal limitations on personal probing. Maybe we should be more suspicious, or at least check quicker on the kind of suspicions I had about Ricky."

"Fine. We're on the same wavelength here, Evelyn," replied Adam. "I would add that once information comes out of the clinician's office, how it is handled is crucial for confidentiality. With the increasing use of electronic records, some experts in informatics—myself not necessarily included—even claim that computerization has the potential to improve protection of sensitive patient information. The banking system had to deal with similar issues of confidentiality, and banks have apparently been able to overcome the stumbling blocks necessary for electronic confidentiality. Even recognizing that a skilled and determined computer expert who has any kind of access might be able to defy our best current security systems, there are still safeguards that The Ethical Way can take, including:

> *"A comprehensive organization policy and procedure for appropriate handling of behavioral healthcare information.* Jonathan Wald recommended this, and I think we should develop one.

> *"Key cards or passwords, similar to the ones used on bank teller machines.* Adele Waller and Jacqueline Darrah recommend that access to sensitive medical information be restricted to authorized users through cards or passwords, and I think it's the least we can do.

> *"Signed statements.* As Randolph Barrows and Paul Clayton recommend, we need another policy and procedure that clinicians, managed care employees, or other relevant people who are granted remote access to patient records will have to sign statements detailing how confidential information is to be processed—and describing significant disciplinary action for omissions.

> *"Match the protection to the level of the risk.* I also like another of Jonathan Wald's recommendations—to keep from chasing our

tails, we need to have graded safeguards depending on the sensitivity of information, ranging from scheduling to patient historical information."

"These guidelines seem appropriate for our company," Evelyn responded. "But if I put my clinical hat on instead of my administrative hat, I'm not so sure how acceptable and relevant they will be for the clinicians we hire or contract with. I think that clinicians will have very difficult decisions to make as to what information is ethically acceptable to share in these transitory times of new managed care systems."

"That is very empathic of you, Evelyn," Sun-Yu responded. "Too many times clinical administrators forget what it was like to be a clinician once they identify with management. And the ethical challenges are different."

"Thank you," Evelyn replied. "I think clinicians should begin with a common traditional process in behavioral healthcare, that being self-scrutiny. Clinicians need to be as sure as possible that their concern about sharing information doesn't stem from their own fears about their treatment being reviewed rather than from their concerns about patient needs. We had to remove several clinicians from our network who would only say that they didn't think it was appropriate to share any patient information with anybody else, since nobody outside the office could judge what was necessary."

"To extend that line of reasoning to the business side," Adam added, "clinicians who protest against using electronic records need to be sure it is not their own computer insecurity or their worry about costs or loss of autonomy that is driving their concerns."

"Good points, both of you," Sun-Yu affirmed. "Then once self-scrutiny is satisfied, the ongoing challenge remains, as Gutheil has advised, to breach confidentiality—even with patients' consent—only when it is as clear as possible that competing goods of more importance would tip the ethical balance in favor of the breach. An obvious example is an acute suicidal or homicidal emergency. More challenging is deciding when sharing information with a managed care company is appropriate, and when it will help to produce cost-effective, medically necessary treatment.

"As an explanation to patients of how such confidentiality questions will be handled, clinicians could provide an ethical code on confidentiality or some sort of written information to patients. To reassure concerned patients, clinicians can offer the patient the chance to review and approve—verbatim—any information that is to be sent out. In fact, managed care companies can insist on using treatment plan forms that require a patient's signature of agreement. Whenever clinicians feel that they cannot meet the confidentiality guidelines of the managed care company, the issue should be discussed with patients for their understanding and approval."

"You know, I encountered a recent example of that," Evelyn added. "A clinician refused to tell our utilization reviewer what the nature and extent of a patient's compulsive behaviors were, saying the patient felt the information was too personal and potentially damaging. Normally, we wouldn't let it go at that, but this clinician usually seems to share information requested and provide cost-effective treatment. I suspect, reading between the lines, that the patient may be a public figure who got into trouble with some sort of compulsive behavior like gambling. I suggested approval of treatment without more information."

"That's not only a nice example of ethical handling of confidentiality by a clinician, but also a helpful trusting relationship between a clinician and a managed care company, to the ethical benefit of all concerned," Sun-Yu commented. "If financially possible, offering complete confidentiality if fee-for-service is acceptable is an alternative. Evelyn, you mentioned how comfortable or not clinicians may be in telling information to a utilization reviewer. I wonder if—"

A lightbulb seemed to go on for Evelyn. She flashed back to the I.C. case—even though it was probably an idiosyncratic, unpredictable confidentiality breach, she decided they should vow in the future to emphasize the importance of confidentiality to all employees, to tell any utilization reviewers how sensitive their position was, and to request only the minimum information necessary to make an authorization decision on medical necessity. She thought another policy change, as I.C. had suggested, would be that the patient had the ethical right of autonomy and informed consent to know the names of anyone involved in their treatment, including the utilization reviewers as well as the clinicians. "Have either of you heard of other managed care companies that have a policy of always telling the patient who is doing utilization review?" she asked.

Sun-Yu and Adam both nodded no, then Sun-Yu added, "But I think it's an excellent idea."

"I agree," Adam said. "And to add teeth to this decision, we can relay to all staff that the company's policy was to fire any staff who breached patient confidentiality outside of company protocol." Evelyn and Sun-Yu nodded yes.

LEGAL POSSIBILITIES

Meanwhile, Sun-Yu again wondered if these complex ethical considerations regarding confidentiality might need some legal standards. With all the major alterations and controversy in the managed behavioral healthcare handling of confidential patient care information, legal guidelines for "which ought not to be voiced about" may become necessary. Legal guidelines may be needed to define which individuals or agencies would have a bona fide need for the information, what information is necessary to share, and how the information is to be protected. She had noted that some states are beginning to produce such legislation—for example, Massachusetts, where a new law stipulates that insurers may only ask for the patient's name, diagnosis, type of treatments, and dates of service.

"Do you think that's enough information, Sun-Yu?" Adam asked.

"Yes, it won't be enough to look at clinical outcomes," Evelyn added.

"Good points," Sun-Yu replied. "Hopefully there won't be too much backlash in the other direction."

BUSINESS VERSUS BEHAVIORAL HEALTHCARE ETHICS SCORECARD

It was apparent to Evelyn and Adam that confidentiality has different meanings and purposes in traditional healthcare and in the business marketplace. Such differences seemed to be an obvious indication for another ethical exhibition game. The scoring rules for who would win were the following:

- *Both healthcare and business ethics win* if relevant and necessary patient information is shared with managed care companies that safeguard the information and use it only to try to improve the quality of cost-effective treatment.

- *Business ethics win but healthcare ethics lose* if managed care companies use patient information mainly to "Monday morning quarterback" and browbeat clinicians just to reduce costs, then carelessly dispose of the evidence.

- *Healthcare ethics win but business ethics lose* if clinicians stand on traditional confidentiality principles and insist that they alone should decide on the best treatment any patient can get.

• *Both sides lose* if integrated healthcare systems can't develop a sense of trust that patient information will be handled sensitively and appropriately between competent clinicians and the fancy new medical information systems.

After shaking hands on these rules, Evelyn and Adam stopped over at the office of their chief financial officer, Buddy Richman, to give him the consultant's bill and analyze any cost implications for the new confidentiality procedures. Buddy winced when he saw the bill and said, "We need to talk about more than confidentiality if we don't want to lose our shirts."

COMMENTARIES ON CHAPTER SIX

As Sun-Yu points out, the burden is on managed care companies to ensure confidentiality. When discussing breach of patient confidentiality, it is important to distinguish between two different types of breach. Confidentiality may be breached either through intentional unauthorized disclosure or through redisclosure of information obtained through a valid disclosure.

Many cases are based on intentional unauthorized disclosure such as the scenario experienced by The Ethical Way. Unfortunately, unauthorized disclosure is simply the result of human curiosity or the desire to use information for personal gain. Many of the ideas to protect confidentiality suggested by the management of the Ethical Way would be successful against this intentional unauthorized disclosure.

The second manner of unauthorized disclosure, unintentional *re*disclosure, is inherent in the managed care system. In the case of unauthorized redisclosure, the information is redisclosed after a valid disclosure; in other words, the patient consented to the original disclosure but not to further distribution of the information. In the managed care environment, the accessibility of information and perceptions of the right to information or necessity for information often lead to unauthorized redisclosure of patient information based on the patient's original authorization to disclose.

Sun-Yu, Adam, and Evelyn generally discuss exceptions to confidentiality requirements that permit disclosure of patient information. Each managed care company should become very familiar with these exceptions because, if not completely understood, improper use of the exception may lead to an unauthorized redisclosure. The exceptions may vary by jurisdiction, facts, and circumstances, and even by disease or treatment being sought by the patient. The key is to understand the limits of the applicable exception so that an unauthorized redisclosure is not inadvertently made by the managed care company.

Several solutions are reviewed by The Ethical Way to ensure patient confidentiality. Following are other ways to protect confidentiality against intentional disclosure and inadvertent redisclosure.

• *Management should question every type of disclosure made to another organization or person.* Each disclosure should be tested against state and federal legal requirements.

• *Management should also strengthen confidentiality requirements in all contracts with payers, employers, and providers.* Contracts should hold the other party to state and federal confidentiality requirements at a minimum. In addition, employers and providers should be held to policies and procedures set by the managed care organization. For example, the employer should have been aware that Ricky's "slip of the tongue" about I.C.'s care should not have gone any further because it was confidential and not an authorized disclosure.

• *A confidentiality agreement should be signed by every employee of the managed care program—not just by the utilization reviewers.* It should be signed again every year to reinforce the employees' commitment to confidentiality.

• *After getting confidentiality agreements signed, the managed care company should continue to reinforce the necessity for confidentiality with all employees.* Enforcement of the confidentiality policies and procedures is a key component of demonstrating an organization's commitment to confidentiality. Patient confidentiality may be a fairly new concept to some employees, who may not have a patient care background. Ricky's comments ("although I'm not functioning as a clinician, I knew it was wrong") illustrate that her knowledge comes from experience as a clinician. Those in the office environment may need to be reminded of the truly confidential nature of the information that they routinely handle.

• *The documents patients sign to release information should clearly state to whom and in which circumstances various types of information will be released.* Valid authorization is one of the best protections against unauthorized redisclosure.

Further, as briefly discussed by the management of the Ethical Way, introduction of the computerized environment provides administrative and clinical benefits but raises significant concerns about confidentiality. The benefits may quickly become risks—computerized records may be easily abused and the nature of the information contained in the records taken for granted. Instituting the safeguards listed here and discussed by The Ethical Way—and periodically weighing the benefits against the risks—will help ensure that appropriate confidentiality precautions are in place and that a computerized system will serve the managed care company to its full potential.

JACQUELINE M. DARRAH, J.D.
Associate General Counsel
Northwest Memorial Hospital, Chicago

The handwritten progress notes of clinicians, historically stored in manila folders in locked file cabinets, are giving way to vast electronic warehouses. The growing data infrastructure and the technological advances in electronic data management have provided healthcare systems with the capacity to integrate horizontally and vertically, synthesize, and use health information with few restraints. Virtual data networks can now link people's health and social service records to all other data collection and storage systems—including those run by the Internal Revenue Service, law enforcement agencies, and the Department of Motor Vehicles. Therefore, people can be tracked and monitored in the most personal aspects of their lives. Most of this has occurred without the knowledge or permission of the recipients of healthcare services.

Recently, when the Kennedy-Kassebaum Healthcare Reform Bill created portability of insurance and more coverage for preexisting conditions, it added at the last moment a provision to facilitate the computerization of medical records in national databases run by the government and private corporations. It will also impose a unique health identifier on everyone so private medical records can be easily accessed. Physicians will no longer be able to guarantee to patients the privacy of their medical records, and the responsibility for developing standards to protect confidential medical records will have been turned over entirely to the Secretary of Health and Human Services. Neither patients nor their physicians will know when sensitive information is released or to whom. Don Haines, on the Legislative Council of the ACLU in Washington, D.C., has warned, "This bill will be remembered by Americans not as healthcare reform but as the thief who stole from us the privacy we deserve for our most confidential medical information."

On the other hand, the development and implementation of managed healthcare plans depend on information about individuals to determine who should be enrolled, to set rates, to determine quality and effectiveness of services, and to engage in prior and concurrent review. Therefore, personal health information has become a refined commodity with considerable worth in the healthcare marketplace. The capacity to transmit patient-specific information within the network of providers benefits patients since care is now integrated through access to computerized information, rather than each episode remaining a discrete, unrelated event.

Still, arguments for public acceptance of such electronic data systems based on promises of better services are not compelling, and issues over access to and confidentiality of health records between providers and recipients have grown over the past few years. In 1996, a CNN poll found that 87 percent of Americans believed that patients should be asked permission every time any information about them is used. It is clear that an improperly thought out and implemented data system can result in invasion of privacy, personal surveillance, abridgment of Constitutional rights, inappropriate monitoring and control of individuals, and access to personal data for private profit or criminal use.

No segment of the population is potentially more vulnerable to these types of violations than those who receive behavioral health services. For people labeled as mental health consumers, the practical consequences of stigma associated with a diagnosis of mental illness can be profound. Inadvertent breaches of confidentiality have precipitated the loss and denial of employment, the inability to obtain housing, and a cascading host of other problems. For this reason, the issues of personal privacy and confidentiality loom very large in the minds of mental health consumers.

At the same time, access to one's own health record to review or make corrections has become increasingly more difficult. The American Psychiatric Association has repeatedly lobbied Congress when health data access and confidentiality bills are being considered, aiming to prevent access to personal psychiatric records if the clinician feels such access is a danger to the person's psychological health. Further, efforts by consumer groups to monitor quality of services and to advocate for patient rights through use of data have also been hindered. Fearing public scrutiny and the loss of enrollees and contracts, managed healthcare companies are claiming proprietary rights of data ownership to control access to information. Often when public agencies and private companies pay for data collection, they demand the right to prohibit the review or publication of health service system information without their permission.

To prevent an escalation in the struggle over access to and security of electronic patient health records, a fundamental change in corporate philosophy is needed. First, the focus on continuous quality improvement of the individual clinician and the service system must be encouraged through the collaborative use of information by all stakeholders in the health delivery system. For consumers, fear can be driven out of electronic data collection by developing participatory action research initiatives, establishing data protection review boards with multistakeholder membership, and building trust and incentives for data sharing. As consumers become equal health information partners and data trustees with providers, they will recognize that even the best systems are not absolutely safe from security failures. Health information partnerships will enable the healthcare industry to move beyond issues of confidentiality and control of health records to embrace the principles of health informatics.

At the core of this approach is the belief that the goals of healthcare data reform cannot be achieved without attending to the way individual health decisions are made. Therefore, healthcare recipients have a right and responsibility to know as much as they can about their conditions, and to partner absolutely in decision making. In direct response to increasing public demand and pressure from government for health organizations to be more open and accountable, a new vision for healthcare in the twenty-first century that is humane, effective, and affordable can be achieved as informed and empowered consumers use the healthcare system more intelligently, with better outcomes, and at significant cost reductions.

JEAN CAMPBELL, Ph.D.
Research Assistant Professor
Missouri Institute of Mental Health, St. Louis

———

This chapter raised several critically important points. However, it failed to stress that the basis of confidentiality rests in the ownership of the clinical record. While various persons may create, enter, or correct information in the record, and while other persons may appropriately access the record, we must maintain our focus on the reality that the record and its contents belong to the recipient of services. When we maintain this focus, it greatly facilitates our ability to deal appropriately with issues of confidentiality.

The focus on policies and procedures in this chapter is necessary, but it will be necessary to create in addition a "corporate culture" around issues of confidentiality. While policies and procedures can create a finite list of what to do and what not to do, it is not possible to anticipate every situation that may arise. If a corporate culture is created, then all employees of the corporation (clinical and nonclinical) will understand that they have a significant role in maintaining confidentiality and that confidentiality is not just the responsibility of someone else. What is being sought here is the kind of individual responsibility for confidentiality that we expect employees to have, for example, with regard to fire safety.

Years ago, when I was responsible for a statewide computerized information system, I was told by the head of the agency that operated the computer center that theirs was a wonderfully secure system. He went into great detail about all of their elaborate security procedures. Two weeks later, I went to the computer center at 2 o'clock in the morning, walked in unchallenged, and went over to the trash can where a computer run with clients' names on it had been thrown away because the run had abnormally ended. I picked up the printout and left with it. Later that day, that agency director and I had a very different conversation about confidentiality and security. Had a corporate culture of confidentiality been created, the computer operator would have known that a printout containing client names didn't belong in an open trash can.

Two other issues that need to be stressed are records retention and information redisclosure. It is important that organizations clarify how long records should be retained. Once a record has outlived its usefulness, destroying it is a significant measure in the protection of confidentiality. Likewise any time confidential information is disclosed, it is important to specify to the recipient of the information what restrictions are placed on subsequent redisclosure. It does little good to be careful about the people to whom you provide confidential information if they in turn are not equally careful with their use of that information.

Beyond these points, in light of the litigious nature of our society, the managed care firm was certainly justified in being concerned about potential legal ramifications from the consumer identified as I.C.

However, the firm created additional liability issues in the way they handled the employee named Ricky. There is significant question whether Ricky should have been allowed to resign, given her complete and total admission of guilt. While this complete admission of guilt may not realistically occur very often, in the context of the chapter the managed care firm probably needed to take more stringent action against her. This error was further compounded when they breached the confidentiality of the employee by telling the consumer the name of the employee who committed the original confidentiality breach.

In terms of I.C.'s request that consumers know who will be reviewing their case, there may well be merit to this request. However, it is important that everyone including the consumers understand that multiple persons may be involved with their data. This reinforces the importance of creating the "corporate mentality" regarding the importance of all employees understanding the role that they play in maintaining confidentiality.

Finally, more discussion on confidentiality and related issues can be found in my monograph, *Confidentiality and the Appropriate Uses of Data*. This document was created through Technical Assistance consultation, which I provided to the Nebraska Department of Public Institutions through funding from the U.S. Center for Mental Health Services. Copies are available through:

> Ronald W. Manderscheid, Ph.D., Chief
> Survey and Analysis Branch
> Center for Mental Health Services
> Room 15-C-04
> Parklawn Building
> 500 Fishers Lane
> Rockville MD 20857
> Phone: 301–443–3343

> ALAN L. ZIGLIN, Ph.D.
> Executive Director
> Northwest Georgia Regional Mental Health,
> Mental Retardation, and Substance Abuse Board

CHAPTER SEVEN

Financial Influences

"Excuse my impertinence," Buddy Richman, the chief financial officer of The Ethical Way, said to co-owners Adam Wilder and Evelyn Bloom, M.D., "but I think it is in the financial area that managed behavioral healthcare faces its chief ethical challenges. And I need to tell you that I think we are beginning to have our own financial ethical challenge right now."

"What do you mean?" Adam asked. "I thought we signed a safe, low-risk Administrative Services Only contract. We're getting 25 cents per member per month, or $300,000 a year, to gatekeep, refer out to a network, and do utilization review on behavioral healthcare for 10,000 people. So where's the problem?"

"The problem is that it looks like we may not be meeting the contractor's financial goals, and our expenses are beginning to exceed our income. The question for us is whether we can adjust some financial aspects without compromising our ethical standards."

"Please be more precise, Buddy," Evelyn implored.

"Well, it looks like the behavioral healthcare cost for treatment by primary care physicians is increasing, when we were supposed to keep it steady. Then the cost of specialty behavioral healthcare by our network of mental health clinicians is starting to edge above the expected $4 per member per month. Now we weren't capitated for those behavioral healthcare costs by either primary care physicians or behavioral healthcare specialists, but our administrative services are supposed to keep that steady or lower the costs. Our administrative costs are also beginning to exceed 25 cents per member per month. We're even beginning to get complaints from clinicians that we're not paying them enough."

"I can see where there might be ethical problems in each of these financial areas," Adam commented.

"Please elaborate," replied Evelyn, "even though spending so much time on financial issues in healthcare still seems odd to me as a clinician."

"Go ahead, Buddy," Adam almost commanded.

"OK, let's talk about the primary care physicians first," Buddy began. "Like in any healthcare system, they provide a lot of behavioral healthcare. Apparently, they are costing the overall system about $3.50 per member per month to do so. The expectation for us is that the costs of their behavioral healthcare not escalate."

"And that seems ethically appropriate for at least two reasons," Evelyn added. "One is that the behavioral healthcare they provide tends to be of questionable quality, so you don't want them doing more until there is some proof of their effectiveness. Second, we could try to refer back to them a lot of the behavioral healthcare done by mental health specialists in the carve-out. That would make the carve-out costs lower, but balloon the primary costs."

"So what should we do with the primary care physicians?" Adam asked.

"I'd suggest escalating the interaction of behavioral healthcare specialists with them to provide more consultation and education."

"By what mechanism that won't cost more?" Buddy asked.

"Well, out of that $300,000 for our contract administration," Evelyn began, "our medical director can divert more time to the primary care physicians."

"And not have the specialist behavioral healthcare suffer, because here too the costs are slightly above the $4 per member per month we're supposed to hold them to?" Buddy challenged.

"Yes, I think so," Evelyn answered. "I think those costs will naturally slowly fall as our network gets used to system expectations and utilization review."

"OK, I can buy that," Adam responded. "If you really feel that $4 per member per month is adequate for the behavioral healthcare to be provided by specialists."

"I think so," said Evelyn. "Maybe not for ideal treatment, everything anyone would want to provide. But it's a working population with apparently little serious, chronic mental illness among the insured or their family members, and comparable populations around the United States seem to have been served adequately for that amount of money."

"Good. You'd better be right," Adam replied harshly. "And what about our administrative expenses out of that yearly $300,000? I can accept some initial loss, as long as I understand why and can see a correction coming."

"Well, I think the problem may be in two areas," answered Buddy.

"One is the management information system, for which we budgeted $100,000 for the year. Although it's still not fully in place, it looks like the $100,000 will be exceeded."

"Oh, that's fine, it's a good investment for the future," Adam replied. "From my previous work, I know how efficient good information systems can be."

"Well, I don't," Evelyn interjected. "I hope that budgeting wasn't at the expense of the more clinically relevant administrative activities, like utilization review. I recall we only hired two reviewers, at somewhat low salaries. We also had trouble with one of them, Ricky."

Buddy started to squirm a bit and said, "Possibly."

Evelyn continued, "I mean, it seems we could have spent a little more on one or both of their salaries, perhaps added another part-time reviewer, and started a little slow with the management information system. Our initial approach sounds like it may have emphasized business aspects over clinical." (And she wondered if Buddy was just trying to please Adam.) "But that approach may have increased costs everywhere if we had poor or overworked reviewers."

Buddy was silent, and after a pause, Adam suggested. "You're making sense, Evelyn. Let's hold off further development of the management information system. Since we haven't replaced Ricky yet, let's spend a little more to look for a more mature, experienced reviewer."

"I'll work on that right away," said Buddy. "We actually have been receiving quite a lot of complaints about our reviewers, especially from clinicians."

"Speaking of clinicians," Evelyn continued. "I have heard they're complaining we're not paying them enough. I thought we were paying the going managed care rates, but trying to do better by them not having any additional withholds on their reimbursement, which would only be paid back to them if we didn't end the year in the red."

"Correct," replied Buddy. "And they do seem to like that. They probably don't like managed care reimbursement rates in general, which in our area is 30 percent below prior fee-for-service rates. More than that, the psychiatrists—and psychologists to a lesser degree—do not seem to like that we have narrowed the reimbursement for psychotherapy."

"Whoops, I sort of forgot about that," replied Evelyn sheepishly. "I knew that wouldn't be popular, but I can't justify us setting reimbursement rates for psychotherapy that would pay certain disciplines so much more than others to provide the same service—not without firm evidence that psychiatrists as a whole provide better psychotherapy than psychologists, or that Ph.D. psychologists provide better psychotherapy than social workers or other master's level therapists."

"Anything you want to try to do about it, Evelyn?" asked Adam.

"I'll talk it over with Barry, our medical director. Perhaps we can set up some meetings with our network providers to discuss our reasons. We can also point out that we do pay more for specialized expertise, such as 10 percent more for psychotherapy of posttraumatic stress disorder."

"What about changing to case rates?" Buddy challenged.

"What's that?" asked Adam.

"Well, that's the newest way to pay clinicians," answered Buddy. "Just give them, say in California, $300 a year to provide all outpatient care per case."

"Only $300 a year!" exclaimed Evelyn. "For a psychiatrist, that would seem untenable. You could probably only do six fifteen-minute med checks a year to feel financially comfortable. Or for therapists, maybe six therapy sessions a year at $50 each would be comfortable."

"But who should determine what should be comfortable?" retorted Buddy.

"Right now, us," Evelyn quickly responded. "And until we get better data on what case rate could produce adequate treatment for particular patient problems or for large groups of patients, I feel we should wait."

"I think we can wait for now," Adam replied. "However, it looks like in this financial arena, we also need further discussion of the ethical challenges, like we previously discussed with gatekeeping, informed consent, and confidentiality. But this time I don't think we need our ethics consultant, Sun-Yu. I think we can use some of her way of thinking, and just discuss it among us three. OK?"

"I guess so," Evelyn answered. "But are we doing that just not to be open with our finances?"

"No, no," Adam quickly replied. "Though that makes good business sense. If I may go on, then, let me tell you both what I think are some of the major financial ethical challenges in behavioral healthcare, then perhaps we can discuss them in more detail.

> "One: the financial ethical issue for the payers of healthcare is whether they are contributing an adequate amount of money for behavioral healthcare.

> "Two: the financial ethical issue for our company—and for other managed care companies—is to survive and use our capital in a way to motivate cost-effective treatment that fits our financial parameters.

> "Three: the financial ethical issue for clinicians is what is appropriate reimbursement for what kind of treatment.

> "Four: the financial ethical issue for behavioral healthcare institutions like hospitals is similar to the one for clinicians: what level of reimbursement is appropriate for hospital treatments and associated administrative costs.

> "Five: finally, for patients or prospective patients, the financial ethical issue centers on how much they should be contributing financially."

"Thanks for the summary, Adam," Evelyn replied. "So it appears that we have a combination of financial ethical challenges. At several layers of the managed behavioral healthcare system, we have the challenge of having the right financial parameters that will enable the desired amount of treatment. In other words, how do we balance and reconcile the costs of treatment with the needs of patients?"

"Yes," Buddy quickly replied. "In the history of health and mental health, there has always been a 'bottom line.' And ethics are not free."

"But we are in a new kind of healthcare system that has not been time-tested," Evelyn quickly added.

A BRIEF FINANCIAL HISTORY

"Speaking of history and time-tested," Adam continued, "maybe you can lead us in a review of how financial influences on behavioral healthcare have been dealt with over time. I know since we first started to put together The Ethical Way that you've been researching and studying this area so that we could learn from history."

"Yes, thanks, I have done that, and if I give a brief historical summary, I think you'll see that managed care seemed inevitable," Evelyn replied, "An article by Joseph English, a recent president of the American Psychiatric Association, reviewed trends in financing mental health services up to President Reagan's time, right before the managed care boom. Let's use that as a summary to give us some perspective."

Evelyn said she'd been surprised to find that in colonial times, financing for mental illness was actually comparatively better than for other medical conditions. The financing was provided by local towns and counties. "To me," Evelyn commented, "the ethical problem at that time in that context seems to have been the repressive approach to patient care, as well as the lumping of the mentally ill with the poor in almshouses."

In the 1800s, the financing for the more severely mentally ill shifted to the states with the development of the state hospital system with medical superintendents. For a long while, the rest of medical care consisted of fee-for-service home visits, with a later proliferation of medical hospitals. "From an ethical standpoint," Evelyn commented, "state hospitals seemed to be an improvement from prior care, though the quality of care seemed to vary quite a bit."

Some fee-for-service outpatient mental health treatment developed in the first half of the twentieth century, before World War II. Much of this stemmed from the growth of Freudian psychoanalysis and psychoanalytic psychotherapy. Because of the fees set by the therapists and the limited numbers of therapists, the therapy tended to be more for the well-to-do. Few psychotherapy advances were applied to state hospital patients, but private psychiatric hospitals emphasizing intensive psychotherapy did emerge. Evelyn felt that here one major ethical issue was the disparity in treatment available depending on social class and financial status.

World War II seemed to stimulate a major change in the provision of psychiatric services and their financing. The high prevalence of psychiatric problems became more obvious, and for the first time, the federal government started to fund psychiatric care. In 1946, the National Mental Health Act provided funds to the states to establish psychiatric clinics, as the federal government had done previously for tuberculosis and venereal disease. Further development of a public health model for mental health led to the establishment of the National Institute of Mental Health and then the nationwide study of mental illness completed by the Joint Commission on Mental Illness and Health in 1961. This led to legislation for the development of community mental health centers designed to serve a much broader population of patients, and also to treat some of the state hospital population in the community, in what came to be known as *deinstitutionalization.* It was hoped that federal support would be only temporary, but the centers did not seem to be successful in obtaining other financial support. Due to the limited numbers of psychiatrists, as well as the preference of many psychiatrists to work outside of such centers, the numbers of nonpsychiatric clinicians—psychologists, social workers, nurses, marriage and family therapists, and paraprofessionals—skyrocketed. The growth of these centers stopped and funding was shifted more to the states starting with President Reagan. Evelyn paused here, with a tinge of sadness as she recalled her days working in the public sector.

"Nice summary, Evelyn," Buddy spoke up, apparently not too comfortable with the emotional aspects of these considerations. "From the managed care standpoint, the ethical issues involved in community mental health may be particularly interesting. How to respond to limited, fixed funding designed to serve a specified population has many similarities to capitated managed care. One major difference, however, is that—at least originally—it appears that community mental health centers were never designed as businesses with the potential to make profits. Moreover, it usually paid to use up all the money you were given by the government, otherwise it would be viewed as unnecessary and taken away. Given the similarities, it may not be surprising that governmental funding agencies, especially the states, are turning to managed care companies to manage and control costs in the public sector previously served by community mental health centers."

Evelyn continued, "Alongside the development of the community mental health centers, various types of insurance coverage for the mentally ill emerged. Federal legislation established both Medicaid (Title XIX) for the poor in 1965 and Medicare (Title XVIII) for the elderly in 1966. Medicare always provided less coverage for mental health services than for other medical disorders. Medicaid funding was geared to each state's per capita income and required some state matching. Reimbursement for psychiatric services, especially outpatient services, was relatively low, and most of the benefits went to inpatient care. These funding decisions are examples of the ethical issue of parity, and whether it is ethically appropriate for less funding to go to the treatment of the mentally ill than other healthcare patients. Not long ago I saw a patient who had $5,000 as lifetime coverage for his schizophrenia, but $5,000,000 for his diabetes and other medical illnesses."

THE INFLUENCE OF INSURANCE

"So where did private insurance come in?" asked Adam.

"That's an interesting history in itself," replied Evelyn. "Private insurance for medical care was originally organized around general hospitals. Both labor unions and businesses negotiated the use of insurance as a nontaxable benefit. Since the mentally ill were generally hospitalized in state hospitals, psychiatric treatment tended to be excluded. As time went on, and psychiatric needs were better recognized and treatment improved, private insurance coverage started to expand. Although the benefits seemed to emphasize hospitalization over outpatient treatment, outpatient coverage in the 1960s and 1970s was enough to greatly expand private fee-for-service treatment, including intensive psychotherapy. Some companies, noted for their benefits, would even pay for most or all of psychoanalysis. States began to mandate a minimum of insurance coverage for mental illness, although here, too, inpatient care was emphasized. States also began to remove the certificate-of-need requirement for new hospitals."

"And that removal sure brought out the financial vultures, didn't it," cackled Buddy, almost salivating. "One major result of this expanded private insurance coverage for mental illness was the rapid development of private, investor-owned psychiatric hospitals in the 1980s. From an ethical standpoint, we even had Frank Rafferty, a doctor who had previously worked in both university and public-sector medicine, make the following points back in 1984:

"He felt that the investor-owned hospital was a morally and ethically neutral component in the development of the healthcare industry in a capitalistic democracy.

"He also felt that the incentive factor of profits for workers, managers, and stockholders in for-profit hospitals was well within the boundaries of American business ethics. He stressed that in practice, the profit system was a welcome and honest alternative to the waste, corruption, and indifference found in some public systems."

"Then maybe we shouldn't be surprised at what happened," Evelyn responded. "Over time, this for-profit hospital development seemed to run into both financial and ethical problems. As both business and governmental concerns about the rise in healthcare costs as a percentage of our country's GNP escalated, it became apparent that mental health costs were rising even more rapidly, up to 60 percent a year, and that private psychiatric hospital costs for adolescents and people with substance abuse problems were a main contributor.

"Later, reported scandals—not everywhere, but there were some big ones in some of the national private hospital systems in some of the states—escalated ethical concerns of overutilization of hospitalization. Concerns over the ethical behavior of providers, especially psychiatrists, revolved around their response to financial incentives that pushed them to hospitalize people and then acquiesce to discharge when insurance benefits ran out—in both cases without much regard to the patient's actual needs. There were even headhunters hired to round up patients for hospitalization. I wonder what Frank Rafferty would think now about how the for-profit hospitals turned out from an ethical standpoint."

"As a quick jump to the present," Adam commented, "it sure is intriguing to me that some of the former for-profit hospitals, at least those who have survived, are now changing their names and trying to turn into managed care systems. I wonder if they've learned any ethical lessons and if we should use them."

"Let's get back to that when we discuss hospitals," Buddy replied. "But I thought it might be interesting to estimate the per member per month costs when those for-profits were at their zenith. For one of the businesses I knew, with a relatively healthy workforce, if you translated the total behavioral healthcare costs that were done on a fee-for-service basis in the late 1980s, it would turn out to be $30 to $40 per member per month! And look what we're dealing with in our contract as a comparison."

THE RISE OF MANAGED CARE

"So given the reduced government support for the public psychiatric sector coupled with the escalating costs and questionable ethics in the private sector, I can now see that perhaps by the 1980s the escalation of managed care was inevitable," Adam continued. Evelyn and Buddy nodded in agreement. "Now if we know what managed care financing has been and what have been the known effects on patient care, then we may be able to say something to our payers about the adequacy of our financial contract."

From the Payer's Perspective

"For management," Adam continued, "funding behavioral healthcare would have to fit into the overall goals and ethics of their business. Generally, I'm sure you'd agree that the goal of any business is to develop a product, be financially viable, and make a profit. One important component to achieve those goals is to have a healthy workforce that will be as productive as possible. Mental well-being should help productivity." (Evelyn nodded vigorously in agreement.) "From a financial standpoint, helping to fund healthcare also makes sense as a nontaxable (so far) fringe benefit for employees and lower insurance rates due to pooling large numbers of patients. Often, small businesses feel they cannot support health insurance by themselves as individual businesses due to limited funds and higher insurance costs."

"A similar process has begun to occur with governmental funding of public-sector mental healthcare. Part of the government concern may be similar to the businesses', which is to reduce costs."

"But doesn't the government also have an ethical and legal goal since it is concerned with a productive citizenry?" Evelyn responded. "We should look back to our country's Declaration of Independence, which read, 'We hold these truths to be self-evident, that all men are created equal, that they are endowed by their Creator with certain unalienable rights, among these are life, liberty, and the pursuit of happiness.' Given these principles, and the relevance of good health for meeting these principles, government should have an additional ethical concern with the health of its citizens. Mental well-being would certainly be particularly important for the pursuit of happiness. In ethical terms, the government would be following the general ethical principle of beneficence, which is for an organization to do all it can to aid patients. Have any financial guidelines evolved to meet these goals, especially in terms of capitation, which is the growing trend and relates to our contract?"

Buddy responded, "Well, the range currently seems to be extensive, from $1 or less per member per month up toward $50 per member per month. The lower figures are more geared to white-collar workers, then the coverage increases with blue-collar, then Medicare, and the highest being Medicaid populations with the chronic, severely ill as part of the population. So a large influence is assumed or known patient need, based on historical patterns. Some of the variation is also associated with benefit level, associated co-pays, the level of local competition, degree of risk, and managed care penetration. Obviously, if the plan spends less than capitation, someone makes money, but if it spends more, someone loses. Various yearly capitated case rates have also been tried on a trial basis with the most seriously ill, ranging in Rochester, for example, from $10,000 to $30,000 a year."

"So we're on the low side with a goal of $4 per member per month, but within that overall range for our mainly blue-collar population," said Adam. "Well, that reassures me somewhat for the time being. So are there any known financial and clinical repercussions from managed behavioral healthcare financing?"

"I can probably answer from the financial side, though not definitely," Buddy responded. "Almost any managed behavioral healthcare plan, whether capitated or not, has claimed cost savings, often initially up to 20 percent. A variety of business mechanisms can be used to control costs, including controls on who can access services, limiting the supply of services, limiting the number of providers, discounted fees for providers, pharmaceutical discounts and formulary limitations, and establishing financial incentives to reduce spending."

"So where's the indefiniteness, Buddy?" asked Adam.

"In a couple of areas. One is it's unclear how long the savings last, given that so many managed care companies are changing and that the public can often change plans yearly. The second area of indefiniteness is whether the savings in the behavioral area are producing increased costs in other areas, such as general healthcare or social costs in lost work time or poorer family functioning."

"Your second point is most interesting from a holistic healthcare standpoint," replied Evelyn, "since there are well-known studies on medical offset costs, where appropriate behavioral treatment results in lowered healthcare costs. Come to think of it, I wonder if we need to educate our payers more about those offset costs. Perhaps that would help them to increase spending on behavioral treatment, especially since it appears that we're having trouble staying in the expected range."

"Let's do that as well as looking at medical utilization when we do our outcome studies," suggested Adam. "We just have to be cautious in pressing for more behavioral treatment, since I'm sure other managed care companies would be glad to assume our financial expectations as they are."

"Or for less," added Buddy, "just to get the business."

"So it looks like managed care financial mechanisms seem to save money," concluded Adam. "How about treatment? Do the cost savings seem to compromise treatment, cause no general change, or even improve treatment?"

"As far as I know," answered Evelyn, "there isn't a whole lot of research comparing managed care to traditional processes, but what is there seems to indicate as good treatment outcomes in managed care, even for the seriously ill. One study of depressed patients did show that the depressed patients of psychiatrists, but not other clinicians, did somewhat worse in terms of functional betterment, compared to depressed patients treated by psychiatrists in a non–managed care system, but the overall improvement in any system was modest."

From the Clinician's Perspective

"Speaking of clinicians, maybe a brief historical perspective would also help us here," Evelyn suggested.

"Make it realistic, Evelyn," Buddy quipped.

"OK," Evelyn started. "I've done some further review on this topic. An idealistic view may be that healthcare clinicians are not in it for the money. After all, they are dedicated to helping others get better, and that is their main reward. Historical evidence, however, suggests otherwise, at least for some clinicians at some times—financial self-interest can also be a strong, and occasionally overriding, motivation.

"Does anything seem different in behavioral healthcare?" asked Buddy.

"Apparently not," Evelyn sighed.

"In behavioral healthcare, similar financial arrangements have taken place. Back in 1967, Ralph Greenson noted the reluctance of psychoanalysts to publicly discuss fees and described 'analytic greed' that accounted for the '45-minute hour' and back-to-back sessions. More recently, *Clinical Psychiatry News* reported that when asked 'What would you do with your profession if you became independently wealthy?' most analysts said they would work fewer hours and 'clear out some dead wood.' (A slight look of horror crossed Adam's face; he had been contemplating trying psychoanalysis. He wondered if an analyst would take him on and then consider him dead wood because of his mild attention deficit disorder.)

Physicians generally charged higher fees for psychotherapy than psychologists, who in turn charged more than master's level therapists or social workers, without any clear data that the higher-paid therapists produced better outcomes. When for-profit psychiatric hospitals emerged, corporate psychiatrists who would do most anything to help fill beds were not hard to find, nor were social work staff to do most of the hospital therapy most cheaply. A recently published study by Mark Schlesinger indicated that psychiatrists have seemed willing to accept more outside constraints and influences on their treatment in return for higher incomes."

"Maybe you're being too hard on clinicians, Evelyn," Adam commented. "From my perspective, it sure appears that most clinicians are much more concerned about providing good healthcare than making money. My guess is that when it appears that physicians or other mental health professionals are more concerned about money, that behavior is unexpected and so contrary to their expected ethics that it really stands out. Buddy, from a business standpoint, do there seem to be any ethical implications on the way behavioral healthcare clinicians have been paid before managed care? Take fee-for-service versus salaried."

"Well, it appears that fee-for-service would offer some incentive to overtreatment, especially if the clinician had schedule openings. It has also tended to produce higher incomes and more clinician autonomy. Salaried positions, which have been more common in the public sector, academics, and hospitals, seem to have different ethical financial repercussions. A salaried position can be a disincentive for necessary treatment, as a clinician still gets paid even when providing less service. On the other hand, possible ethical benefits for salaries are known costs to the payers, clinical teamwork and mutual monitoring, and common continuing education."

"Go on to the changes produced by managed care," Adam suggested.

"A variety of changes in reimbursement have been tried for behavioral healthcare clinicians," Buddy continued, "including:

"Discounted reimbursement rates for seeing managed care patients, 20 percent or greater, occasionally with added discounts withheld in case the company doesn't do well. (Providers really hate these, as they're often never paid.)

"*Limited payment authorization* for services only when they were approved as 'medically necessary' by the company's own utilization reviewers, resulting in significant amounts of unreimbursed treatment whether through missing or unapproved treatment plans.

"*Emphasizing medication over psychotherapy* by paying psychiatrists more for time spent in prescribing medication than in psychotherapy. The difference can be really dramatic, such as $30 to $50 for fifteen-minute med checks compared to $90 to $100 an hour for psychotherapy.

"*Forming closed networks of providers* who have to agree to the payment mechanism and processes, while only paying 50 percent or less to providers out of the network.

"*Bonuses for reduction of specialized services.* Bonuses show up most often in salary contracts in a capitated system of care."

"The obvious thrust of these financial strategies is to reduce costs by lowering fees, motivating less treatment, and reward certain kinds of treatment over others," Adam commented. "These seem to be sound, ethical business strategies to me, but what do you think about them from the ethical perspective of a clinician, Evelyn?"

"They've left me and other clinicians with many ethical challenges, among them:

"Is it acceptable to participate in these systems of reimbursement?

"Will these financial incentives and disincentives adversely affect treatment?

"What is a satisfactory income level for the work produced?

"Will you decide to make clinical decisions based on sound research findings and assume that cost-effective care will be an inevitable consequence?"

"What sort of response or results have you seen to these challenges?" asked Adam.

"Certainly we have seen more than adequate numbers of mental health clinicians join and accept the managed care financial parameters, although a groundswell of opposition is forming," Evelyn began. "Though certain kinds of treatment are being emphasized, such as psychopharmacology, brief psychotherapy, and brief hospitalization, it is unclear whether overall patient care is being compromised as a result. Interestingly enough, there have been few ethical complaints lodged against clinicians using this kind of treatment emphasis. Salaried managed care clinicians are being paid well, while those who freelance and see patients under a variety of payment mechanisms are having much more variable financial success.

"In one survey done by the National Association of Social Workers, social workers had the highest rate of income increase—12.7 percent-among the mental health disciplines over three years in the early 1990s. This increase occurred despite more involvement with patients under managed care and a slightly lower fee reimbursement under managed care. Another finding of the survey was that direct payment from patients was the primary source of income for social workers and counselors, whereas psychologists and psychiatrists reported third-party payers as the prime source of income. Since we're talking about clinicians here, does anybody know the difference when tables are turned, that is, when clinicians are owners of the managed care system?"

"Apparently so far that hasn't been much different from when non-clinicians own the company," Buddy replied. "Even under clinician-led managed care systems, financial needs seem paramount. And, to me, our financial needs are paramount now. From all this discussion, it seems like our business strategy to control expenses makes ethical sense as far as clinicians go. But if not, is there anything more we can do about clinician reimbursement?"

"Let me answer first in general," Evelyn replied. "I have been grappling with these ethical challenges since we thought of forming The Ethical Way, but once we got started, the challenges and concerns of running a company also affected my perspective. I think I've gone from wanting to protect clinicians' financial status, rights, and independence to a more balanced viewpoint incorporating other perspectives."

"We're waiting," Buddy said half-demandingly and half–good naturedly.

Evelyn replied, "I was about to say that I've come to the conclusion that payment for clinician services needs to be based on one factor: treatment benefits. If the basis of healthcare ethics is the care of the patient, how well a clinician does that should be the determinant of reimbursement, not necessarily degree, experience, history, rhetoric, or reputation. Presumably that would also make business ethical sense since patients would do as well as possible with less wasted time and effort."

"Makes perfect sense to me," said Adam. "So why isn't anyone doing it—including us?"

"Well, the challenges to obtain the relevant data are enormous," answered Evelyn. "Even putting aside individual patient variation, just getting accurate data on how a given clinician does with various types of patient problems has been formidable. Often, a clinician will get a certain reputation of excellence in general or for certain kinds of patients, but without any sort of verification. We're just now—thanks to managed care, I think—developing the kind of instruments that can provide ongoing monitoring of treatment to predict and document its benefits. Once this process becomes more sophisticated, we and other managed care companies can pay the better clinicians more, adding even extra payment for the most difficult patients, and I bet we'll save money."

"I won't bet against you. So what do you think, Buddy?" asked Adam with an air of support for his partner.

"Well, it does sound promising, and I think most anybody would like to know that their clinician had a proven track record of success," Buddy replied in a conciliatory manner, "and we do pay more for better lawyers, better universities, and better cars."

"Good, and it would certainly behoove any clinician to do everything possible to document quality of care" Adam concluded. "One more type of clinician we haven't discussed here is students. We're about to start using them in the network of clinicians that we're managing, but maybe we should cancel that now since I've heard they're too expensive for managed care organizations."

From the Student's Perspective

"It seems like we have another financial and ethical challenge with students," Evelyn resumed. "Let's look at the changes. Until recently, the education of students in the mental health disciplines has been financially supported through a variety of mechanisms, but with payers making the main contribution. Financial support also included faculty supervision time and related expenses, as present in Medicare 'pass-through' support. Since students often received their training in the public sector, the federal government has been a major contributor.

"Although many have stated that educating students costs much more than the services they provide are worth, it seems that conclusion may apply only to medical students. It looks as though graduate mental health students do provide a lot of potentially valuable treatment. Most people don't know about Barbara Lerner's study from the 1960s, which showed that in providing psychotherapy to the poor, student interns often produced better results than experienced clinicians. I also wouldn't be surprised if we someday found out that resident psychiatrists at times did better than psychiatrists in practice in prescribing newer medication."

"That could fit your plan to pay those who do the best no matter their experience," Adam added.

"Thanks," replied Evelyn. "For the faculty who teach students, reimbursement for their time was usually assumed to be subsidized from clinical work, research grants, or administrative funds. With the rise in managed care, the contribution from clinical work may be threatened. One recent study by Steven Shea of a department of medicine in a prominent medical school found that teaching time is poorly compensated, at a rate of about $16 per hour excluding fringe benefits."

"Sixteen dollars an hour even seems too low to me," said Buddy.

"Do you know how managed care organizations have tended to respond to this issue?" Adam asked.

"Yes, and the response has been a little mixed and somewhat contradictory," Evelyn responded. "Managed care has not only affected the payer system, but has raised questions about financial support and clinical participation of mental health students. On one hand, although there have been a few managed care settings that have emphasized student education, many managed care companies will refuse to pay for the clinical or educational involvement of students, even on a fee-for-service basis, and will imply that quality is improved because students are not used. On the other hand, managed care companies have been critical of academic institutions for not producing clinicians familiar with managed care principles. To top all of this discussion off, I'll have to admit that it appears that some academic institutions have been guilty of financial fraud with Medicare overcharging and inappropriate use of research funds."

"Any suggested solutions for us here?" asked Buddy in a less challenging tone.

"Yes, and we don't necessarily have to compromise cost-effective managed care principles in the process," Evelyn continued. "The challenge with students is for managed care companies to support their education in managed care in a—here's that phrase again—cost-effective manner. For example, we could include psychiatric residents, psychology interns, or social work students by expecting them to be able to pay for their stipend and supervision by doing a certain amount of clinical work."

"Pay them how much?" Buddy interrupted.

"That's the key," Evelyn replied calmly. "If we pay them only, say, half of rates for their counterparts in practice, that should take care of their stipend, even allowing for a third of their time to be spent in educational activities. I'm sure you could calculate the figures more precisely, Buddy."

Buddy was already working on his calculator and started to nod in agreement.

"Of course, even if we and possibly other managed care companies accept the use of students, we'll need the cooperation of residency and other educational directors. Linkages and cooperation with academic institutions to develop appropriate stipends and quality assurances will be important to train future clinicians in managed care principles. Academic centers themselves will need to accept managed care more than they have, try to develop some of their own managed care programs, and adapt their educational programs accordingly. Managed care companies are also beginning to experiment with starting their own residency and intern educational programs."

"OK, we can do it," Buddy looked back up. "I mean, at least to support stipends. And we might be able to save up to one-third of clinical costs if the students provide beneficial treatment."

"So this is another way we can potentially save money in the future. Anywhere else we should look?" asked Adam.

From the Hospital's Perspective

"What about hospitals?" Buddy suggested. "Just as with our network of clinicians, it's been up to us to pick which hospitals we'll use and how much to pay them. We didn't discuss changing hospitals or reducing rates to them."

"We can review that, Buddy," Evelyn answered, "but first let's put hospitals in a broader perspective. Hospitals used to be a high-cost item. But what a change the last ten years have been for hospitals! Whereas for-profit hospitals did quite well financially for a while when certificate-of-need was removed, indemnity insurance devoted more coverage to hospitalization than outpatient treatment, and hospital rates were paid in full, the tides have often turned with managed care. As managed care authorization has reduced so-called unnecessary hospitalization and dramatically reduced length of stay—and negotiated discounted packaged day rates much less than half of customary charges for stays they did authorize—psychiatric hospitals and units in general hospitals have suffered financial stress. At times, managed care companies seem to have just pitted hospitals against each other on the basis of cost. Many hospitals have closed or consolidated. Staffing patterns are tighter and certain adjunctive services like recreational therapy reduced. About the only hospitals that haven't been affected in this way are those that have directly entered the managed care marketplace, either by offering their own managed care products or forming physician-hospital organizations to do the same. The operational results are still usually a reduction in beds and an expansion of traditional inpatient beds into day treatment, outpatient, and even residential services."

"Very interesting," commented Adam. "It seems like hospitals have really been on the cusp between business ethics and healthcare ethics. From the business side, it appears that they have charged whatever the market would bear, and did quite well in the 1980s. On the other side, they've had a tradition of developing healthcare ethics codes, which we previously discussed, and at many times had a reputation for good patient care, but have run into ethical, legal, and financial problems in recent years. It will be interesting to see if they can develop and maintain some leadership positions in the managed care marketplace."

"It looks like they, too, whether for-profit or not-for-profit, are renaming themselves to present a new image, calling themselves healthcare systems or the like," Evelyn replied with a hint of skepticism.

"Yes, it looks like the managed care bandwagon is attracting all kinds of interest," Buddy added. "But The Ethical Way is not hospital-based, so we're probably getting astray. Hospital-based companies, though, do have one financial advantage compared to us. If they have extra beds, they can cheaply absorb the hospital costs instead of paying a per diem or case rate like we do to hospitals we contract with."

"And the discounted rates to hospitals probably can't go much lower and our length of stays are good, so there doesn't appear to be much else to save here," concluded Adam.

From the Patient's Perspective

After a pause, Buddy began again, "You know, it's curious that we haven't yet discussed the possible ethical financial responsibilities of those who are benefitting from treatment, the patients."

"Yes," replied Evelyn. "I guess it's because under our current contract we can't do anything about patient payment. We have no co-pays and no point-of-service option. But it is important to discuss for future possibilities. It appears we have backtracked from the bioethical principle of patient autonomy here. But maybe we're getting ahead of the story for patients. How much patients should pay for their mental health treatment has varied over time and circumstances. In 1980, patients paid for 35 percent of all mental healthcare. Self-payment is much less or none for the indigent, even though some would argue that some meaningful co-pay would make the treatment itself more meaningful. Moreover, a hard-liner might maintain, why should treatment be subsidized for those who can spend money on street drugs? On the other hand, Gregory Simon found that increasing copayments has been found to decrease demand in a progressive manner regardless of severity of illness. There is also a magic number of $7 co-pay a month." (Adam and Buddy looked confused.) "It seems that patients are loyal to their physicians until they have to pay more than $7 per month, and then they tend to move on. Except for the wealthy, that is, who even if they could afford to, do not usually pay more than standard fees.

"Psychoanalytic psychotherapy has tried to incorporate payment and participation as part of the patient's overall psychology, so that missed sessions are billed for as therapy sessions since they are part of the ongoing therapy and have important meaning. The American Psychiatric Association's Code of Ethics has been worded in a way to allow this practice."

"Is that similar to the rest of medicine?" Adam asked. "I don't remember ever being billed by other physicians for missing an appointment."

"It is somewhat different, Adam," Evelyn answered. "As an example, if a patient misses an EKG, the physician may bill for a missed visit but not the EKG. Psychoanalysis, in this financial conception, is more like bundled surgical services. Extended to other, less intensive psychoanalytic therapy, billing is considered part of the treatment for which the patient's responsibility for payment is important."

"And how has managed care responded to these traditions?" Buddy again challenged.

"Managed care financial practices seem to be altering the responsibility of patients for direct payment, as well as obfuscating some of the background financial processes," Evelyn began to respond. "In the newer capitated plans, patient co-pay is none or negligible. There may be no fee negotiation exposed, or even allowed, between provider and patient. If there is a point-of-service plan, and if the patient does go outside the designated network, then patient responsibility for payment escalates, often to 50 percent or more. The concept of bundled psychoanalytic sessions, or reimbursing for missed sessions, has generally not been accepted by managed care companies. Again, the financial incentive seems to be to use the managed care plan and accept the practices of the plan. If savings or profits are made, this doesn't seem to lead to more services or lower premiums to the consumer."

"And how do you think patients are being affected by these changes?" Adam asked.

"How much patients seem to understand about the financial ramifications of their managed care mental health coverage is unclear," Evelyn replied. "There seems to be no principle in place that advocates extensive education for patients before or when they obtain managed care mental health coverage. Patients themselves may not know what they are missing, and if they don't feel a financial obligation, they may tend not to ask."

"While we don't have the option to charge patients in our current contract—and I wish we could—what would you suggest, look for, or advocate for the future?" Buddy asked.

"Although never definitely proven, I would tend to agree with psychoanalytic tradition and indemnity insurance with co-pays that assume that there is some value for patients to make significant financial contribution for their mental health treatment if they can manage it," Evelyn responded. "Maybe that is less relevant for the rest of healthcare, but for behavioral healthcare the intertwining of psychopathology and finances indicates that some financial responsibility by patients could actually be therapeutic for them. In the very least, patients should have a clear understanding of the financial parameters and processes of their managed care plan. When patients pay for treatment, they not only know all the financial parameters, but may recognize the potential conflict of interest for the clinician in getting paid more when doing more. The patient could ask for or obtain a second opinion when in doubt. One unusual strategy might be to find ways for patients to participate in the capitation process."

"How so, Evelyn?" Adam asked. "After all, we can't put patients at risk financially as they're already at risk for their mental well-being!"

"Well, perhaps as one possibility, for certain high-cost patients who are not very compliant with treatment, they could be offered a percentage of savings if they are more compliant, do better, and save the system money."

"Fascinating," Buddy responded, "though I suppose that unusual strategy will need further consideration."

Evelyn and Adam both agreed, though they didn't want to be the first managed care company to try something like that.

BUSINESS VERSUS BEHAVIORAL HEALTHCARE ETHICS SCORECARD

Later, Adam and Evelyn mused over these complicated financial ethical considerations. By its operating practices, managed care has changed many of the financial practices and influences on mental health treatment.

While many of the separate components of these practices have been done before, including reimbursement reductions (in Medicare and Medicaid) or limited services due to overall budget limitations (in community mental health centers), the entire package seems to be unique in its controlled and managed approach to reducing costs and unnecessary treatment.

In a bioethical sense, this is taking an extreme paternalistic approach by in effect stating that the managed care company knows what is best for both clinicians and patients, and that's all it will pay for.

In a healthcare ethical sense, less and less financial autonomy is left to clinicians and patients. Managed care companies have used legally binding contracts to ground this approach. In the process, if large savings or profits are produced for the payers and managed care companies and not necessarily funneled back into healthcare, that is consistent with business ethics.

Besides the process for managing the money, how much money is appropriate for a given mental health managed care system to manage has only developed by trial and error and how much the market will bear. The amount of money is usually either similar to the prior costs, or—in the case of capitation—to the prior sums minus a small percentage. For mental health, such an approach is especially questionable, given the amount of care provided by primary care physicians, the traditionally lower spending in the public sector, the different fees charged by different disciplines for the same treatment, and the documented extraordinary numbers of people who need treatment but do not seek it.

The current ethical challenge is to define the appropriate financial responsibilities for payment of behavioral healthcare services and the appropriate distribution of those payments. If the question is who should profit and by how much, the ethical answer may still need to take into account how much potential patients will "profit" in their care as a result of such decisions.

"So are we now ready to move on?" Evelyn finally asked.

"Not until we agree on another ethical exhibition game," Adam replied with a touch of competitive edge.

"Again? All right, but what sort of scoring rules can we use, given the variety of business, governmental, clinical, and citizen parties involved?" Evelyn asked.

"How about this?" Adam revealed some notes he'd made.

- *Both healthcare and business ethics win* if we maintain the profit margin we've chosen and there is some overall improvement in the quality of care while unnecessary harm (actual and potential) to patients and providers is assiduously avoided.

- *Business ethics win but healthcare ethics lose* if managed care companies produce large savings or profits for themselves and the payers, but there is a reduction of overall quality of care so that large numbers of patients suffer needlessly and good clinicians are prevented from participation in the system.

- *Healthcare ethics win but business ethics lose* if clinicians endeavor to provide the ideal and best treatment (psychoanalysis and long-term hospitalization is potentially available to all) and bad clinicians are ignored, so that healthcare costs continue to rise, some patients get dramatically better, and some patients don't improve or worsen despite extensive treatment.

- *Both sides lose* if payers decide they can no longer afford to support mental healthcare, so that only the rich can try to find the good clinicians and bare warehousing is available for the poor.

As they shook hands on this competition, the phone rang. "Guess what?" Adam said with a grin when he hung up. "We won the bid for a full-risk capitated Medicaid contract in New County, Central Carolina." This time they hugged in mutual congratulations.

"Now we can really get into treatment issues," Evelyn concluded with some excitement.

CHAPTER EIGHT

Treatment

$\mathbf{I}$sn't it amazing that we have spent so much time and money discussing ethical issues that are not directly involved with patient care, which to my mind is still our primary mission?" wondered Evelyn Bloom, M.D., co-owner of The Ethical Way.

"Maybe it's only amazing that those sorts of issues were not addressed more in the past," the other co-owner, Adam Wilder, commented.

"You mean cost-effective treatment?" asked Evelyn.

"Partially that," answered Adam. "Although if cost wasn't a societal concern at times, perhaps that wasn't always a major ethical issue. You showed me past healthcare ethical codes that didn't mention cost issues, except for not charging unreasonable fees, not fee-splitting, and paying some attention to societal needs. However, one could make a case that the two or three-tier behavioral healthcare treatment systems we've had before managed care posed an ethical problem."

"In what sense?" asked Evelyn with interest.

"Well, patients in the public sector like community mental health surely received less and different treatment than those with good indemnity insurance, who surely received less than wealthy patients who could pay for whatever they wanted," Adam responded.

"So you think patients always received different treatment depending on their financial status," Evelyn reflected. "That seems true for the most part. Patients in the public sector were much less likely to receive intensive psychotherapy than those with good insurance or ability to self-pay who had the same problems. Often, the more you were covered financially, the more treatment you received."

"Plus there was so little monitoring of treatment effectiveness," Adam continued. "Clinicians essentially did whatever they wanted, without guidelines, dependent only on the patient's compliance, as important as that may be. Normal narcissism would leave most clinicians feeling that they had provided good treatment."

"And now that we've got this new contract, we'll need to see if our management can provide as good or better treatment," Evelyn added. "Any updates on that contract?"

"Yes, that's really why I asked to talk to you today. We're hard at work on the capitated carve-out contract for New County, Central Carolina—the state accepted our bid two weeks ago and there are still some implications and procedures we haven't thought through. We have an at-risk partnership with a community mental health center. Other bidders were community mental health centers alone, local managed care companies alone, and national managed care companies. Besides this contract being a joint venture, it is also different from our last one in that our system will be at full risk financially instead of just managing services for a fee. It appears that our joint bid was most competitive in terms of finances, and your experience in the public sector and our concern about ethics also helped win it. Maybe the state also thought a joint private and public venture could meld the best of both. We will receive about the same amount of money—$30 per member per month—that was spent in the system last year. The higher capitation reflects that this serves a predominantly indigent multicultural population with a large percentage of the more seriously and chronically ill. The contract is for five years, a length that will allow us to get to know the population covered well and provide continuity to those chronic patients needing long-term treatment. To begin, one of our big challenges is to develop a common systemic culture that will combine the old values of community mental health and managed care."

"Yes, I remember from my days in the public sector," Evelyn replied, "that community mental health seemed to be provider-oriented to the extent of adding more staff to try to provide more services to those in need, even if they couldn't afford it. Also, the accountability to community boards, the state, and the federal government made change cumbersome."

"Whereas managed care tends to be focused on what precisely is in the contract and likely to move quickly," Adam added quickly. "Those differences are reflected in how we've set up the initial administrative structure. To reduce unnecessary costs and keep a managed care orientation, most of the administration of the community mental health center was let go. Board members were asked to serve on an advisory board, which of course would not have the same authority as previously. However, we decided to keep their clinicians, feeling they were used to providing treatment under limited financial parameters."

"However, those clinicians do not seem to trust our business orientation, so putting in a more managed care focus on treatment will likely not be easy," Evelyn concluded. "We might want to increase our administrative case conferences for a while to process how we're doing."

"Agreed," agreed Adam.

TREATMENT PLANNING

Evelyn and Adam, along with their medical director, Barry "The Bear" Grayson, had began to discuss what general principles could be used to guide them toward cost-effective treatment with this new contract. The first step in cost-effective treatment would be appropriate treatment planning. To do so, they would have to take into account the guidelines given by the state. To keep costs near their current level, the state designated that a managed care approach needed to be used. The basics of the approach included:

- Use of a multidisciplinary staff
- An average of ten psychotherapy visits a year of any appropriate modality, continuous or intermittent
- An average of ten brief medication checks a year, individual or group
- Consideration of costs in choice of medications
- Case management services as needed
- Review committee approval prior to more intensive treatment
- Outreach to patients who don't keep appointments
- Reduction in hospitalizations

Reviewing these principles, Adam and Evelyn asked Barry if he saw some immediate ethical issues that would affect treatment planning. After thinking for a while, Barry replied, "Well, I don't have too many problems with the overall guidelines for numbers of sessions and medications, since the numbers of sessions a year fit national average outpatient visits and we have flexibility for more depending on individual needs. Any good managed care program should reduce hospitalizations, so that shouldn't be a problem. The interesting ethical issue to me, though, seems to be the use of the multidisciplinary staff."

"Why would that be a problem?" asked Adam. "That seems to be a reasonable expectation."

"It is," The Bear growled slightly. "The ethical problem is, how do we decide who does what the best, not only from a disciplinary standpoint, but also from an individual competence standpoint? There is still so much variation in what behavioral treatment is provided for the same problem. Then there is the legal issue of credentialing. Sometimes community mental health centers will have hired staff who are not necessarily licensed by the state. Finally, I wasn't sure whether they meant 'multidisciplinary staff' to allow inclusion of consumer or family representatives."

"You mean to hire consumers?" Adam asked a little incredulously.

"I wasn't exactly thinking that," Barry responded quickly, "although consumers have been hired and done well in paraprofessional positions, and of course many substance abuse counselors will have had a history of recovery from substance abuse. No, I meant if we were going to follow our ethical guidelines of informed consent and patient choice, that it's become well-known that consumer involvement and input is important for the care of the more chronic, seriously ill. Moreover, since their problems often have such a strong impact on families, those family members, including local representatives of the National Alliance for the Mentally Ill, should be involved in some ethical way."

"What would you suggest then?" asked Evelyn.

"Well, if we're planning to have an administrative case conference, let's invite consumer and family representatives to get their perspective on how we're doing," Barry suggested. "How about John Channing, a patient with schizophrenia who has done well and is working, and Freddy Famelletti, a family member active in the Central Carolina Alliance for the Mentally Ill?"

"Sounds good," Evelyn replied, "as long as we disguise the identity of any patient discussed for confidentiality."

"Right, so we'll invite them," Adam agreed. "It will also be interesting to see how the clinical staff is reacting to the system change and the new managed care treatment approach."

AN ADMINISTRATIVE CASE CONFERENCE

Before the administrative case conference was to be held, a treatment plan was sent out to all the main participants for the case to be discussed. "You mean all these clinicians are involved in this one case?" Adam asked with some surprise. "The treatment plan is signed by Stacy Goode, a social worker, but also involved is the psychiatrist Sam Citron, the psychologist Seth Moody, the nurse Nancy Singer, and the paraprofessional Polly Blackman. What did we get into with this Medicaid managed care contract? I'm getting second thoughts already. I hope all the cases aren't like this."

"No, don't worry about that," Evelyn replied. "This looks like an unusual case, but one reason it was picked is that it touches on many important ethical treatment issues and involves representatives of all the disciplines. So we can probably all learn a lot from this case that we can generalize to other patients. Here's the brief summary."

The patient, Jane Doe, is a thirty-four-year-old African American woman. Jane came into the treatment system almost a year ago with a diagnosis of schizoaffective disorder. She did fairly well until about three months ago when her mother, whom she lived with, died. Since then she seemed to be withdrawing. She reported worsening auditory hallucinations with self-critical content, and she was losing weight. She attended her usual treatment appointments, had a monthly medication check, received monthly Haldol Decanoate shots and the antidepressant imipramine, and also received supportive psychotherapy once a month.

Her history indicated multiple hospitalizations since late adolescence. She had been able to go to school or hold a job only briefly. There had been intermittent substance abuse, which often preceded hospitalizations.

In childhood, she had seemed fairly normal until about age ten, when she started to withdraw. From then on, she became more overweight and particularly uncomfortable around men.

"Interesting case, so what are they asking for in the treatment plan?" Adam asked, ever ready to move on.

"It looks like they want so much they ran out of space on the form," laughed Evelyn.

"Yes, consider all of this," The Bear grumbled a bit:

"They would like Seth to do some psychological testing to clarify the diagnosis.

"They would like the medication evaluations by Sam to increase to weekly.

"They would like Nancy to be able to make a home visit if Jane misses her appointment.

"They would like Polly to perform some case management services, including locating alternative living possibilities.

"Stacy, who completed the form and has coordinated Jane's care, would like to increase her supportive therapy visits to weekly."

"Well, obviously we need more information before we authorize all this," The Bear continued, "including more of their reasons for why this would be cost-effective and how much time is to be spent in each treatment session. It ought to be an interesting conference. By the way, one first-year psychology student, Izzy Wolf, is attending."

Psychological Testing

They held the conference in the mental health center conference room, to emphasize that the center was the clinical fulcrum site. It was located at the fringe of the inner city, with somewhat cramped quarters, old furniture, and the best views being of the parking lot. Not exactly like the modern, high-tech administrative offices of The Ethical Way, Evelyn thought to herself, with some hope that they would improve the facility if they were financially successful. The participants included all staff involved in the treatment plan, other center staff, consumer and family representatives, and some administrative personnel. The Bear decided to start with the request for psychological testing, since that seemed so unusual in the days of managed care.

"So, Seth, why are you asking to do psychological testing and what do you want to do?" The Bear demanded. "After all, the patient has been diagnosed over the years. What could testing possibly add now? Jane just seems to be grieving her mother's death and her symptoms are intensifying. Besides, testing is so expensive."

"Well, apparently her presentation seems readily explainable, but there also seem to be some subtle but important diagnostic considerations and questions," Seth began. "For instance, since she's been in treatment so long, has the schizoaffective diagnosis just become a wastebasket for her? There is a slight hint of early sexual abuse, so has that been missed? Are her current symptoms more suggestive of a worsening thought disorder or depression? What sort of therapeutic approach would be most valuable at this time?"

Izzy was the first to respond to the questions. "I can't believe we're even discussing whether or not to do the testing. Doesn't every patient have the right to the best evaluation possible?"

"Perhaps in the best of all worlds, Izzy," The Bear snapped. "But if we did everything we could to make as sure as we could be, there wouldn't be anywhere enough money to go around to pay for such comprehensive evaluations. And in a capitated system like ours, if we do too much traditional testing, we'd definitely lose money. Besides, maybe a skilled clinician could tease out these issues."

"Besides balancing Jane's treatment needs and costs, are there any other ethical issues here?" Evelyn questioned. "It's particularly interesting to me why psychological testing has come to be used so infrequently in managed care."

"I've grappled with this issue before in other managed care settings," The Bear replied. "And one particular ethical principle in the Code of Conduct for psychologists always has struck me. In Standard 2.07, Obsolete Tests and Outdated Test Results, it says that psychologists should not base their assessment or recommendations on tests that are outdated or obsolete for the current purpose. So, Seth, do you have any tests that have been updated or revised to fit a managed care setting?"

Seth seemed caught off-guard and impressed. "You mean, you've actually taken a look at our Code of Conduct? I hardly know any psychologists who really examine what's in there, let alone a nonpsychologist. We just seem to have a general impression of what's in there."

"Until an ethical question like this arises," Barry smiled, The Bear moving into the background. "Isn't that an ethical problem in itself, that most of us—no matter which discipline—really aren't familiar with what is in our professional ethical codes?"

"I suppose you're right," Seth conceded.

"But that doesn't help us to decide what to do in this case," Evelyn responded. "Is there psychological testing adaptable to this case, Seth?"

"Actually, I think so," as Seth relaxed a little. "In preparation for our system changing to managed care, I tried to catch up on the topic and ran across a very helpful recent article by Kevin Moreland—'How Psychological Testing Can Reinstate Its Value in an Era of Cost Containment.' Possibly helpful in this case would be multiscale psychopathology inventories like the MMPI–2, SCL–90–R, and PAI, which could help assess complex problems. These tests can even be helpful to distinguish between internalizers or externalizers, which in turn can help predict whether patients will benefit more from insight-oriented or supportive psychotherapy, respectively. Since we're thinking about increasing therapy sessions, the Therapeutic Reactance Scale can help determine whether Jane will readily follow Stacy's therapeutic suggestions."

"Sounds helpful," Adam reacted. "But as our chief financial officer would ask—and maybe he should be at these conferences—how much will this cost? After all, one reason such batteries have not been authorized in managed care settings is that they typically take seven hours and cost an awful lot. They can use up most of a patient's outpatient coverage when that coverage is limited to a state mandate, say $1800, although we don't have that limitation in our capitated contract."

Seth replied, "I've tried to look into that—one way we can save time and money is through the use of computers."

"Are you ready to do that?" The Bear demanded.

"Not quite," Seth quietly responded.

"Then work on it and get back to me before we decide to use the testing in this case," The Bear concluded. "For now, the testing is not authorized due to high cost and the likelihood we can get most of the same information from sound clinical assessment."

"I'll help you, Seth, if you like," offered Adam enthusiastically, thinking of how he might apply his software background.

How Much Treatment

After some grumbling and nods of approval in the audience, Barry went on. "So let's go on to the treatment requests. You all know that sometimes no treatment is the treatment of choice, right?"

A look of disbelief swept through some in the audience, especially Izzy Wolf. Izzy was even thinking that the treatment plan was not asking for enough. Maybe even day hospital or inpatient treatment would be the best.

After a pause, Barry smiled a little and said, "No, I'm not talking about Jane here. But we should realize that there are times when no treatment would be the ethical treatment of choice, not to just save money. Can you think of any criteria for no treatment, Izzy?"

Izzy had started to think about that. "Well, some of the patients who were court committed for treatment never seem to get any benefit," he said.

"That's right," Barry replied, "although it is interesting that many of them do get better and even turn out to be grateful. In general, we can look at three categories for no treatment:

"First, those patients likely to have spontaneous improvement, such as developmental reactions to unexpected events, including deaths. Even with Jane, we should clarify how much of her reaction is normal grief. It seems that at least 10 percent of patients improve spontaneously after calling for an appointment.

"Second, those likely to have no response, such as antisocial personality disorders or malingerers.

"Third, those at risk for a negative treatment response, such as patients with masochistic or severe narcissistic traits."

"Anyway, in this case it certainly looks like treatment—even more treatment—is necessary, don't you think?" asked Stacy. "Jane is really suffering now and can't do much of anything."

Treatment Readiness

"I agree she needs treatment, and perhaps more as you've asked for. But is she ready for treatment?" The Bear asked. "Here, too, managed care has stimulated further consideration of when a patient is likely to benefit from treatment. In a comparable community mental health center, the psychologists Robert Raskin and Jill Novacek found three behaviors that indicated a lack of treatment readiness: Repeatedly missing appointments, not talking about relevant problems during sessions, and inability to recognize warning signs of decompensation."

"And what happens if these behaviors occur?" John softly asked. "I mean, some of that used to apply to me."

"And to my son," chimed in Freddy. "How is this new managed care system going to address these behaviors? Just let someone like Jane fall by the wayside?"

"No, we're expecting to make their treatment even better. Without governmental restrictions and bureaucracy, we can do some innovative things," Adam said assuredly. "We can bring some of the spirit of invention that I found in the software industry."

Polly then added her paraprofessional perspective. "I'm looking forward to this change," she said. "At first, I was skeptical about managed care, that the companies would just rip off the people for profits. But then I read about the experimental program in Rochester, New York, where a patient a lot like Jane was released from a brief hospitalization. Right away, the case manager was able to use undesignated dollars to pay a security deposit on an apartment and pay for groceries and other essential supplies."

"That's exactly the flexibility we want," Barry smiled. And we'll have that financial flexibility if we're careful about treatment readiness. Getting back to that, the Raskin and Novacek study we began to talk about also showed how much money could be saved by addressing treatment readiness."

"How much, so we can tell Buddy, our chief financial officer?" Adam asked.

"Just consider these consequences," Barry said. "Those patients who missed three or more appointments cost an extra $1,500, or almost 30 percent more per patient to treat over an eight-month period than the ones who stayed in treatment and followed recommendations. The patients who did not talk about their problems cost even more, an extra $2,300, or 44 percent more. And the ones who were unable to recognize their own signs of decompensation cost an extra $1,800, or 33 percent more.

"And besides using more money, how did these patients do?" asked Freddy.

"Not surprisingly, not too well," commented Barry with a sigh. "Those patients ended up with more severe symptoms and a poorer quality of life, at statistically significant levels."

"These patients were probably difficult for staff, also," Stacy said.

"Yes, that was actually the last finding. Those patients ended up being viewed by their clinicians as more difficult to work with and taking more time."

"But you still haven't told us how you'll address this unreadiness, as you put it," John reminded everybody.

"Well, we'll try to follow the recommendations that came out of that study," Barry responded. "To avoid missing appointments, use all the usual reminders, but also use beeper technology." (Adam's eyes opened wide at this plan.) "To help patients talk about their problems, educate them as to what they should talk about. And for recognizing decompensation, develop 'help-seeking skills or groups,' in which patients work on simulations of when and who to call for help."

"It sure sounds good," Freddy responded. "But the Alliance for the Mentally Ill has heard nice promises before, and been disappointed."

"You won't with us," said Evelyn assuredly. "How about if we look now at Sam's request to see the patient weekly?"

Medication Monitoring

"Sam, the weekly visits for now seem indicated, maybe even more until Jane seems to improve, but you didn't put down how long you wanted to see her each time: fifteen minutes, thirty minutes, or even more?" Barry asked. "I hope you're not completely against fifteen-minute med checks."

"No, I'm not, although I enjoyed the article by William Houghton, M.D., which wondered whether Freud would have approved of them," Sam calmly replied. "Of course, we tend to forget that Freud did a lot of brief therapy, even on walks. But with Jane, until I can decide what medication adjustments are needed, I'll likely need at least a half hour. I'd also like to keep Nancy involved, since she's gotten to know Jane so well through providing her shots. And, if we can't get Jane in, I'd like to go with Nancy to make a home visit. I assume home visits are a possible authorized treatment."

"You're right," said Evelyn. "Just like with day treatment, managed care seems to be provoking a revival and enhancement of some old innovations from community mental health, including home visits. In fact, having a nurse's aide stay at home with Jane at $10 an hour could be more cost-effective than hospitalization."

"OK, that sounds like a good medication plan," concluded Barry. "And I'm glad you didn't mention hospitalization."

"Well, sometimes nowadays getting into a psychiatric hospital is harder than getting into Harvard Medical School," Sam quickly quipped.

Psychotherapy Planning

"I am, though, more unsure about the psychotherapy plan you asked for, Stacy," continued Barry after a brief smile. "Wouldn't it be more cost-effective and meet Jane's needs to have Sam or even Nancy just attach on some psychotherapy to their medication contacts? After all, so far we really have no firm research as to whether medication and therapy are better done by one person or split."

Looking at first hurt, then angry, Stacy blurted back, "Doesn't my prior relationship with the patient count for anything? You managed care companies just come in and throw therapists away as if we were old cars. Especially older therapists, because you can probably get the younger ones cheaper. If you do anything like that, I'm going to tell the patient and complain to your ethics committee, if you have one, or to the state," she went on.

"OK, OK, it was just a question, maybe more rhetorical than otherwise," Barry backed down. "Since the optimal relationship with schizophrenic patients is so crucial, and it appears that you have that kind of relationship, your therapy requests are authorized. For now, anyway—but the authorization is only for one month, then you should be ready to meet less often again since Jane should be over her crisis by then. Please submit a new treatment plan then."

Case Management Services

"OK, and if I caught your implication before, case management by Polly is also authorized," Stacy went on with a little hesitancy. "You must realize that case management has a different sort of tradition in community mental health than in managed care."

"Yes, we do," Evelyn added to the discussion. "I recall from my own experience in the public sector that case management involves a variety of activities to address any problem area in a patient's life, whereas in managed care, case management is usually done behind the scenes, with a distant relationship with the patient, to monitor the medical necessity of treatment and control the use of resources. Due to the importance of the relationship in the public-sector type of case management, Polly seems ideal, not only from her extensive experience and training, but also being of the same ethnic background as the patient."

"Yes, thanks, Evelyn," commented Adam. "And if we add the managed care type of case management, we can add the ethical business needs to supplement the healthcare ethics we've been discussing." (Adam thought to himself that although they were authorizing a good part of the treatment plan, much of that was relatively cheap and might help to avoid higher-cost services like hospitalization.

Besides, community mental health clinicians should be used to limited options.)

Treatment Teams

"So it looks like we're all set with the treatment planning in this case," Barry concluded, "and it looks like you're a good, smooth-functioning team. About the only clinician we haven't discussed is the primary care physician, but I gather from the absence of medical problems on Axis III, as well as the sophisticated medication issues, that the primary care physician is not needed at this time. We do, however, have to be alert to any possible indications of medical problems, which tend to get overlooked in these kinds of patients."

The team nodded in agreement.

"And I assume you all are willing to work evenings and Saturday morning, and be available after hours for calls," Adam added. "After all, the treatment needs of patients don't confine themselves to eight-to-five."

"Right, and I'm sure you'll agree that it is ethically appropriate that we charge for such services, and that maybe it shouldn't be for straight-time rates," Sam the psychiatrist reacted.

"Yes, as long as it's medically necessary," agreed Adam.

"Great, so it now looks like we're all ready to go on to discuss the treatment process when we meet again next month," as Barry was ready to end the conference.

"Just one minute," one of the new utilization reviewers piped up. "I notice the treatment plan is not signed by the patient. Doesn't she agree?"

"Yes, but since we were unsure of what your response would be and how you'd handle informed consent, we decided to wait until after this meeting to have her sign," Stacy the social worker quickly responded.

"Fine, everything's open to tell the patient, depending on her needs," Barry concluded. "See you all in a month."

THE TREATMENT PROCESS

Between conferences, the mental health center clinicians shared their doubts in informal meetings in the halls. While they agreed that so far The Ethical Way seemed ethically better than most managed care companies, and they were pleased by the authorization of most of their treatment plan, they wondered how The Ethical Way would react to some of the treatment they thought was ethically appropriate. Did The Ethical Way participate in the growing practice of removing Zoloft from the formulary, since Sam the psychiatrist was ready to make the switch to Zoloft from imipramine? Would they agree to pay for the more expensive Clozaril or Risperdal, as the benefits of Haldol Decanoate seemed limited? Would they continue to authorize psychotherapy beyond twenty visits a year? Would they pay for special group activities like celebrating ethnic holidays? And would they support nonverbal creative art therapies for the more guarded patients? Sam would bring up his concerns in the next conference—other issues would be brought up by staff when it seemed clinically relevant to patient care.

On the other side, The Ethical Way administration was fairly impressed. Though the team was asking to do a lot, they seemed flexible, accepting of cost-effective principles, and willing to be reviewed.

Meanwhile, back at the psychology intern training site, the faculty seemed split on Izzy's report of his experience. Some were aghast to hear that Izzy was being exposed to limited treatment before knowing ideal treatment, and to the subtle bias against psychoanalytic psychotherapy. Others felt that the jury was out on the pros and cons of managed care, and that their academic center should become more involved with managed care and participate in outcome research. For now, they would wait to see how Izzy's educational experience progressed. They continued to process among themselves their diverse views on managed care.

One other place where the conference was processed was the monthly meeting of the local Alliance for the Mentally Ill. Much anxiety was present, as John and Freddy still wondered if The Ethical Way wasn't really more interested in money than in them. But they were impressed that the company seemed more open with information and more flexible than others they had heard about.

Prescribing Medication

"I'm glad to see everybody back," Barry began the second monthly administrative case conference centering on the patient Jane Doe. "Some time has now elapsed since the initial treatment planning, so let's see how Jane is doing. Since there is so much we might talk about in her treatment, let's focus on ethical aspects of the treatment—The

Ethical Way wants to pride itself on its ethics. So, Sam, let's begin with her medication treatment and particularly discuss two cost-effectiveness issues, medication checks and choice of medication. Let's start with the nature of the med checks—you weren't sure how much time they would take initially, and there really isn't any research that compares the effectiveness of fifteen-minute, thirty-minute, or longer checks with weekly, biweekly, or longer intervals for patients with comparable symptoms."

"Well, using the managed care way," Sam responded with a little sarcasm, "I tried to keep the medication reevaluations as brief as possible. Actually, that seemed to fit Jane's psychology at the time—she had become more quiet and withdrawn, and not as conversant as before. And I am following Barry Blackwell's recent recommendations on how to do a brief medication check: establish a relationship by asking about real, everyday experiences, by emphasizing how medication can help quality of life, and by connecting the medication to other treatments. But we did need to meet more often, twice-weekly for fifteen minutes, as we were changing two of her medications. Now, as she's beginning to improve, I'd like to meet with her for half an hour weekly until she is stable again," Sam continued. He almost choked on using "like to," which was a change from his usual "plan to," as if he was asking the managed care company for permission to treat his patient. After all, he was just asking for authorization for payment, as he had decided he would do what he thought necessary whether it was authorized or not since Jane was in crisis. But he realized he couldn't do that with most patients or he eventually couldn't earn a living. "We don't have those twenty-visit limits per year, do we?"

"No, not for crisis situations, though we're trying to average ten fifteen-minute medication visits a year per patient for financial stability," Adam commented. "From the data we received on prior treatment of many of these patients, that should be enough."

"So you're OK here for now," Barry continued. "But I expect that she'll be stable in a month and you'll be back to monthly visits. So you're authorized for a month and then you should send in a new treatment plan to our utilization review staff. And what sort of medication changes have you started and why?" The Bear began to challenge.

Barry had come to believe that most clinicians tended to lean toward providing extra treatment when in doubt, not usually for financial greed, but because of a long-standing ethical tradition to put the patient's needs first and to do no harm. He felt his job and that of managed care would be to balance that tendency to overtreat, so that instead of "when in doubt, do," a principle of "when in doubt, don't" would evolve. What made these decisions so ethically difficult was the lack of firm guidelines of what to do with an individual patient. He felt that perhaps as little as 20 percent of behavioral healthcare practice had a firm scientific basis that could be applied in an individual case. Then, thinking of Jane specifically, he knew that controlled clinical research trials had rarely studied combinations of medications, let alone how much the different medications might cost. Suddenly Barry realized that Seth had begun his response.

"Since Jane's prominent symptoms were those of depression and she had been on the tricycle antidepressant at adequate doses for so long, I felt a change was warranted in that one of the newer antidepressants might be more helpful. So I picked Zoloft, assuming that it was on the formulary."

"Why Zoloft? There are many other new antidepressants," Barry tried to ask in a neutral way.

"For one, because I've had a lot of experience with it and seen its success. Then I also like what I'm hearing about its characteristics compared to the other new SSRIs. For instance, new studies indicate that Zoloft can be stopped for a day or two and sexual responsiveness will return if that is a side effect. Also, it seems to have less interaction with other medications."

"Those reasons seem appropriate, though more research needs to be done," Barry responded. "And, by the way, Zoloft is on our formulary, in part because state regulations require all medications to be available to Medicaid patients, whereas managed care companies serving non-Medicaid patients can determine their own formulary. We also feel that it could be unethical that some managed care companies have removed Zoloft from their formularies when they are using a pharmaceutical benefits firm that is owned by the makers of one of the competing medications, Paxil or Prozac. The firm makes formulary decisions and negotiates prices with pharmacies. But what about costs? Did you consider that?"

"No, I can't say that I did, nor have ever, unless patients told me that they couldn't afford one of the more expensive new antidepressants," Sam responded.

"And I suppose that you never told a patient that the new antidepressants could be just as cost-effective as the old, so in the long run a new one would likely be as cheap," the Bear challenged. "Why are you so blasé about costs? Is it because the community mental health center just used whatever money was available?"

"Well, I am concerned about costs in the sense that I feel good treatment will be best for costs in the long run," Sam responded. "Anyways, it sounds like it's authorized for us to use Zoloft."

"Yes, it is," Barry replied, "but only because the cost-effectiveness studies have been inconclusive so far. One study by the pharmacologist David Sclar found that the old tricycle antidepressants like Jane was on cost $366 a year more per patient compared to Prozac in one large network-model HMO. That sure makes it hard to accept the policy of some large managed care companies that require a failure of two old tricycles before the use of something like Prozac. Sclar also reported in another study that Prozac seemed to be slightly more cost-effective than its newer rivals, Zoloft and Paxil. But then you have another study led by Thomas Einarson and conducted by an independent group of university-affiliated investigators from a number of disciplines. Here they found that in an inpatient setting the new serotonin norepinephrine reuptake inhibitor Effexor demonstrated the highest level of cost-effectiveness when using both brand and generic acquisition costs of the comparative SSRIs, old tricyclic antidepressants, and a heterocyclic antidepressant (trazodone). In the outpatient setting, however, trazodone was the most cost-effective, though in terms of just effectiveness, the SSRIs had the highest success rate. Finally, in one study in a primary care setting, Paxil was found to be as cost-effective as imipramine."

"Well, I'm just glad Zoloft is still available," Sam commented, "and I'll be anxious to see if my own personal preference turns out to match the research. And maybe the pharmaceutical companies can help out by reducing the cost of their medication. But I am confused about what that term 'cost-effectiveness' really means."

"Me, too," responded John right away.

"Me, too," followed Freddy, followed by nods in most of the audience.

"Do they teach you that in your training program?" Barry asked Izzy.

"No, they try to teach what's best for the patient," Izzy responded with pride.

"And damn the costs. It's the ivory tower way," The Bear growled. "Well, if that attitude doesn't already hit your school in its pocketbook, it will."

"It is an important question, Barry," Evelyn interjected. "Just what does this cost-effectiveness mean in terms of prescribing medications?"

After a bit of stammering, Barry responded, "You know, after reading all the rhetoric by the managed care companies and the scientific literature, I'm still not sure. If we separate out costs, that's the easy part. Costs generally include acquisition cost, medical care, laboratory tests, and side effect management. Effectiveness is more complex and can be looked at in a variety of ways, such as symptom-free days, quality of life, likelihood of achieving minimal effective dose, time of onset, and prevention of relapse. But cost-effectiveness and how to combine the two is really confusing. The key ethical question is how to decide on how much effectiveness is relevant at what cost."

"Well, I'm glad there's still some uncertainty here," Sam continued. "Because we have the same consideration with Jane's neuroleptic medication. I decided to try a switch from the Haldol-Decanoate injections once a month to the new Risperdal pills for the possibility of better effects on her negative symptoms."

"That sounds like a reasonable clinical judgment, Sam," responded Barry, "but over time we'll also have to look at the costs of noncompliance, side effects, and that the medication itself is more expensive. Overall, I'd like us to keep the formulary open—new studies are starting to show that limiting medication choice may cost more in the long run."

Psychotherapy

"Let's look at Jane's psychotherapy now," Stacy continued after a pause, wanting to get her part over with. "My, I thought medication considerations would be simple compared to psychotherapy, but maybe it's the other way around, at least in Jane's case. I mean, you know the cost of my sessions and there's very little likelihood of side effects."

"But just like there's a wide variety of medications, there's all kinds of psychotherapy, and treatment goals can be pretty vague," countered Barry. "That's one big reason why we have treatment plans that need to be redone at any change in treatment or at the request of the utilization reviewer who decides whether the requested plan would be authorized and for how long. It is especially important to provide a justification for the planned treatment. All clinicians should try to follow the credo of James Sabin, who maintains that it is ethically mandatory to recommend the least costly treatment unless there is strong evidence that can be cited that a more costly treatment is likely to produce a much better outcome."

"Granted," Stacy responded. "I've tried to be cost-effective by seeing her less than I might have before, and done it in conjunction with her medication visits. She has been involved, seems to be beginning to mourn her mother appropriately, and is starting to look at other living situations."

"Thanks for trying to adjust your practice, Stacy," Barry replied. "As the saying goes, 'try it and you'll like it.' Other therapists have tried to be more cost-effective and found it acceptable and not unethical. Managed care is also spurring the development of new instruments that can monitor the progress of therapy as it proceeds. I hope you'll be agreeable to such monitoring, Stacy."

"Of course," Stacy replied with a sweet smile. "That would be the ethical way."

The conference was running out of time. They briefly touched on the case management services Polly provided to help update the patient's finances, as well as new transportation needs, all for the cost of two traditional psychotherapy sessions by psychiatrists. They adjourned until the next conference, which was moved up to two weeks hence.

DISCHARGE PLANNING

As the next session of the case conference began, to discuss treatment termination, The Bear opened with a challenging statement to the treatment team, "I hear that Jane just went into the hospital."

"Let me explain," Polly offered. "It was a surprise to us, too. Someone from the hospital called our emergency number after a neighbor called the hospital. Jane was apparently up in the middle of the night, yelling and throwing things. I went over there with the police to see what was going on."

"You went over there in the middle of the night," Barry repeated, impressed.

"Yes, to try to see what was going on—and to try to avoid hospitalization," she added with a smile. "I found what looked like cocaine around and Jane later told us an old friend brought it over. Since we didn't know it at the time, we brought her to the hospital for safety and to try to find out why she decompensated."

"Now that you did, is she ready to leave?" Barry asked.

"Not quite ready, I feel," responded Sam. "Now she's more despondent at what she did and feeling suicidal. So I don't want a twenty-eight-day AODA program, but I would like a day or two more to reduce her guilt and for Polly to talk to that so-called friend."

"OK, so you can have one day only, and if more seems needed, how about the in-house nursing aide or day treatment?" Barry suggested. "This plan would fit our use of the medical necessity scales for inpatient care."

Feeling reassured that The Ethical Way really did try to balance healthcare ethics with business ethics, Sam agreed. He was relieved he wouldn't be faced with an ethical and legal dilemma of not receiving authorization for payment, having the hospital press for discharge, but being unsure that the patient was ready. *It's really hard sometimes to know when to take a risk of discharge or not,* he thought. He also felt fortunate that alternative services to inpatient care were available.

"So we're in agreement about hospital discharge. Do we have any expectations about outpatient discharge?" Barry asked. "Please, no hesitancy—I hope by now you all realize we aren't the kind of company that will punish you for advocating for your patient treatment needs. On the other hand, if we ever come to a difference of opinion that can't be resolved immediately, we expect you to not leave patients without an appropriate source of care."

"Are there any legal standards to fall back on in such disputes?" Izzy asked nervously.

"Not exactly," answered Barry. "Of course, there is malpractice law, but that is flexible to a degree on relying on local professional custom, so that in a community that is shifting to more managed care, professional customs of treatment may not be obvious. We as a company realize that we also have the potential to be sued if we don't respond expeditiously and objectively to timely appeals. If there's still disagreement with the appeal decision, we have an ethics consultant to use. I hope later that the state government will set up a patient review board with no conflict of interest as a last appeal process. Anyway, I'd be surprised if there's any major difference of opinion about future treatment for Jane."

With some hesitancy, Stacy responded and said, "It seems like Jane has the kind of complex and serious disorder that will require outpatient treatment of some degree indefinitely. To anticipate stopping that, or even to mention that possibility to Jane, would likely put her at risk for decompensation."

"Agreed," Barry said. "And we hope you'll be able to continue with her during that time. Continuity of care will be especially important for her. Just keep costs in mind, especially if we have many more patients like her."

John and Freddy whispered to each other that they were surprised, but that it looked like The Ethical Way was as devoted to patient care as patient costs.

"Our time is about up for today. At our next conference on Jane, let's consider the treatment issue of outcomes. Even though we are not planning on Jane's discharge, outcomes are important to consider both during and after treatment."

OUTCOMES

By now, Izzy was becoming more positive about managed care, at least this managed care. He was coming to see that maybe the ethical goal of treatment could not always be the ideal treatment under any circumstances, but at least it should be adequate treatment that fit the healthcare system's financial parameters and the needs of other patients. He appreciated learning to provide a spectrum of treatment for similar problems. And he was looking forward to the discussion of outcomes, especially from an ethical perspective. He had been taught research skills but not outcome skills.

Barry began the next conference with a question. "Why are we even talking about outcomes in an ethics-oriented conference on a patient who is not likely to be discharged?"

Seth, who had been quiet since the psychological testing on Jane had been put on hold, seemed interested in the answer. "If our ethical goal is cost-effective treatment, how will we ever know if the treatment is effective if we don't do outcomes? And I think there are some simple measurement tools that can be given to the clinicians and patients that will verify our outcomes, outcomes for The Ethical Way as a whole, but also to find best practices as models to follow. Can The Ethical Way pay for that?"

"Yes, we've begun with a reserve pool of 2 percent to be used as seed money to begin outcome studies," Adam answered.

"And can I include Izzy as part of his intern stipend time?" Seth asked.

"That should be an ethical use of our capitation money," Evelyn concluded, "since it has the potential to improve patient care and involve students in the old Hippocratic tradition."

BUSINESS VERSUS BEHAVIORAL HEALTHCARE ETHICS SCORECARD

Evelyn and Adam were finding these administrative case conferences to be a cost-effective use of their time. They were really getting a good sense of the real everyday ethical challenges the clinicians and administrative staff met. And despite the financial risk of the new capitated Medicaid contract, they felt confident as the community mental health team seemed to function like a finely tuned musical ensemble. They accepted their different roles, were flexible, could overlap if necessary, and seemed to have an open mind about managed care. One of them had commented after the last conference that although there seemed to be as much bureaucracy in managed care as in the traditional public sector, at least managed care was forcing the group to try new treatment strategies and talk more about the ethical issues involved in cost-effective treatment.

They did, however, realize that this was an ethical game they could lose, so they once again decided on criteria for whether they would win or lose.

- *Both healthcare and business ethics win* if healthcare costs were better controlled and treatment outcomes improved.

- *Business ethics win but healthcare ethics lose* if costs were better controlled, but patient outcomes worsened.

- *Healthcare ethics win but business ethics lose* if outcomes indicated patient care improved, but the costs were unsustainable.

- *Both sides lose* if the new managed care systems only produced temporary cost savings and temporary improved outcomes, or sustained cost increases and quality-of-care reductions.

Both realized that appropriate utilization review would help them win, but that The Ethical Way seemed to be having some problems in this area. One earlier key employee, Ricky, had to resign. They had hired more new reviewers for the new contract, but they had been strangely quiet at this administrative case conference. Perhaps they now needed to hire a chief utilization reviewer.

—〰—

COMMENTARY ON CHAPTER EIGHT

Mark Twain said, "Always do what's right. It will gratify some and astonish the rest." This chapter on treatment attempts to explore ways in which changing forms of treatment delivery have brought into question centuries-old ethical traditions. It provides some overview of the ethical dilemmas that are encountered and ways of thinking ethically so as to feel on a morally justifiable high ground. It takes as a fundamental proposition the need to balance business and professional ethics. It also takes a fundamental position that the clinician or administrator of a health plan can adequately balance the needs of an individual patient, the needs of a group of patients, and the needs of the professionals who rely on payment from that group for their sustenance.

Having experienced and been asked numerous questions about maintaining professional values in the midst of dramatic healthcare change, I believe it is fair to say that the situation is not quite as simple (nor as complex) as presented. There has to date been no mental health professional organization that embodies the extent of the principles as articulated. Indeed, if we examine the principles I am most familiar with—those of the American Medical Association (AMA) and American Psychiatric Association (APA)—there would be some areas of overlap but many areas of disagreement.

Where then do the ethical dilemmas as articulated in this chapter, the principles advocated, and the principles of the professional organizations converge? First, the AMA and APA state unequivocally that the physician's primary responsibility is to the care of the patient and advocacy for the patient whether as the primary treating clinician or as administrator. Does this mean that we should advocate always for ideal or marginally beneficial care? No, we should advocate for care that is materially beneficial to the patient. We should follow guidelines for patient care that are based on scientific evidence. When there is no such scientific evidence, judgment and prudence must be applied to determine appropriate treatment. When there are two types of treatment with the same outcome, the less costly intervention should be used. Indeed, it is unethical to knowingly provide unnecessary care. However, when it comes to the question of giving slightly more care or slightly less care, my perspective would be to provide more care if the outcome is uncertain. Although I greatly respect Dr. James Sabin's opinions, I disagree with him in this area. Sometimes we can't have absolute scientific evidence to make a determination. It is especially repugnant if delivering less care increases the amount of reimbursement for the clinician, thereby placing him or her in a conflict of interest.

The chapter rightly points out the need for flexibility in treatment decisions. A standard forty-five- or fifty-minute hour is not a prerequisite. Continuity of care is highlighted, as is judgment in use of medications unfettered by pharmaceutical maneuvering. Clinicians should be in a position to prescribe and treat in a manner that is scientifically valid and in the least restrictive environment. Unfortunately, in this case vignette, I would think that the patient would not be fully informed of all the discussions regarding cost-effectiveness of various treatment approaches. If there really was respect for patient autonomy, there should be full disclosure.

It is important that these questions are raised, that different ethical positions are highlighted, and that professionals decide which ethical positions will have longevity in our society. In my view, healthcare ethics should win, with the result that society will need to make informed allocation decisions. Dr. Sabin and I agree that a single-payer system may provide the needed justice in our currently fragmented and unjust system and would mitigate many of the concerns I have raised. I congratulate the author on attempting to sort through these thorny issues and opening up his book to commentary. This is in the true spirit of scientific and ethical discourse.

JEREMY A. LAZARUS, M.D.
Associate Clinical Professor of Psychiatry
University of Colorado, Health Sciences Center

CHAPTER NINE

Utilization Review

A s The Ethical Way grew, Evelyn Bloom, M.D., and Adam Wilder decided they needed to hire a chief utilization reviewer. In developing criteria, they chose to begin each interview with a variation of a joke that was going around. That way, the interviews could be short and sweet, in the managed care manner.

Apparently there was a short line at the gates of Heaven waiting to meet St. Peter. First in line was a community mental health clinician whom St. Peter asked, "How was your stay on Earth?"

"Hard, but morally rewarding. I took care of a lot of those in need, but didn't make anywhere as much as my colleagues in private practice."

"Come on in," answered St. Peter. "You did God's work and you can stay here indefinitely."

Next was a child psychiatrist. "I did my best for those kids, but it sure was hard, having to also deal with parents, schools, and even the court system. Over the years, I've seen many of them overcome their problems."

"Welcome," St. Peter responded. "What can be more God's work than helping unfortunate children?"

Next was a managed behavioral healthcare utilization review director. "I, too, helped others, St. Peter. Not only patients, by only authorizing them to get what they needed, such as reduced hospital length of stays—you know that nobody likes to be in the hospital—but I helped justice in society by controlling healthcare costs."

"And also made even more for your company and yourself, and didn't turn any of it back into healthcare, correct?" asked St. Peter.

"Yes, but that's the American business ethical way," replied the reviewer.

"Well, I guess we can apply that same managed care criterion here for you, then," replied St. Peter. "You're authorized to stay here for three days."

"But what is that? Another kind of gatekeeping? I want a second opinion. Is God around?"

"That's all the time available to you. Next . . . " (The reviewer was then dragged away protesting his authorization by a former clinician he had denied.)

What Evelyn and Adam were looking for was some kind of mixed reaction, laughter but also concern. They thought of utilization review as the atomic energy of behavioral healthcare, something with enormous power that could be used for either destructive or constructive purposes. The destruction could be quick like an atomic bomb, eliminating good providers and good treatment wholesale under the guise of cost savings. Or the destruction could be slow and insidious like radioactive fallout, contaminating the whole behavioral healthcare system. This is how Evelyn felt—perhaps from her biased viewpoint as a psychiatrist—about the policy of many companies to not authorize psychiatrists to do outpatient psychotherapy. At its constructive best, she knew, utilization review could offer a balanced second opinion to consider the goals of payers, insurers, clinicians, and patients.

Their chief financial officer, Buddy Richman, was also looking for a flash of anger when their candidates heard this joke, so that denials wouldn't be too hard to give. Buddy was given hiring authority since utilization review had such important financial implications.

They quickly went through a lot of candidates who did not respond to the joke as they desired. Then they met U. B. (for Ulysses Bradley, but always called U.B.) Wright. He was a clinical psychologist with a background in researching treatment results and many recent years as a utilization reviewer. And he responded to the joke as they had hoped.

"Well, if I got there for three days, I'd use them effectively to give St. Peter some pointers," U.B. laughed. "Including how much money those do-gooder clinicians were possibly wasting that could go to the care of others really in need," he added with some indignation. "Then I'm sure I'd be authorized for a longer stay." That he had been a champion debater in high school added the likely bonus that he would be able to handle—and usually win—any arguments with clinicians.

Starting with gusto, U.B. was swift and efficient in his denials. He thought that was what Buddy wanted and felt justified. There would be no long-term psychotherapy for panic disorders, as obviously medication should do the trick. Children with conduct disorders would not be authorized for hospitalization for their parents' convenience. For suicidal depressed patients, three inpatient days and you better be out.

Any suspicious treatment plan necessitated a full chart review before authorization. And, of course, no psychoanalysis would be authorized, even if it was provided at a low fee that would fit under the benefit limits. If he received too much protest, U.B. would sweetly say, "I'm only denying authorization for payment. Of course, you can—and should if you're worried—continue treatment, for you are responsible for that." And if they still disagreed, he'd paint an ominous picture of appealing to their medical director, Barry "The Bear" Grayson. He was finding it easier and easier to "just say no!" So although they had an appeal process to use the medical director when clinicians disagreed with lack of authorization, U.B. tried anything he could to divert that process so he would look good. None of the higher administrators heard any complaints and Buddy was happy with the cost savings.

A CASE EXAMPLE

Then one day Adam and Evelyn heard from Barry, their medical director, who had gotten a call from the mother of a patient. It had to do with the case of a young woman who complained of having trouble concentrating after developing some sexual interest in a new male friend. This was the first time as an adult that she had such sexual feelings and she was surprised by them. What was striking from her evaluation history was a report of sexual abuse by a male cousin in his early twenties when she was about ten to thirteen. She said that memories about the sexual interactions had always been with her and she didn't feel too bothered by them, except for the cousin telling her she was so ugly. She turned out to be quite overweight and was eating even more now. She had told her mother once, as the abuser was the son of the mother's older, much-loved sister who had helped to raise the mother. The mother seemed not to have believed the patient when the patient told her years earlier and apparently hadn't done anything about it at that time. U.B. had denied any treatment at all, unbeknownst to them. His written notes indicated that he felt there was no question that this case lacked medical necessity at the time since the patient seemed to be functioning pretty well. Evelyn then asked Adam if he agreed with U.B.'s decision.

"Well, I'm not a clinician," Adam answered, "but it sounds to me that this was just the tip of the iceberg for this patient and if we didn't do something to help now, she'd probably need more help later. And consequently cost us more."

"Agreed," responded Evelyn. "Also it seems like the patient's functioning was compromised by being unable to develop an intimate relationship with a male and starting to lose focus, which could jeopardize her job (and as she said that, she silently wondered if Buddy and U.B. would like the patient to lose her job—or die—so she would lose her insurance and they no longer would be responsible for her). To be sure, there might be some disagreements among clinicians and reviewers involved about what treatment might be best for this case. Some might think that just supportive, brief therapy would be enough to help the patient go on with the relationship. Others—perhaps especially women—would think that more intensive, insight-oriented therapy was necessary to help the patient make connections with the earlier reported abuse so she should feel less threatened and more in control for any future relationships with men, and maybe also resolve some lingering resentment to her mother that was coming out in overeating.

"Again, this feels out of my realm, but it would seem that in the long run, her insurance dollars would be best used to provide as definitive a therapy as we can under the dollar limits of her policy," responded Adam.

"I also agree with you," replied Evelyn. But here we are with both of us recommending definitive therapy, but our new chief of utilization had authorized nothing."

Barry continued with the patient's history for Evelyn and Adam. Apparently, the man the patient was interested in turned out to have a criminal history of rape, which the patient knew but hadn't had time to tell the evaluator. Frustrated at her slow response, he raped her, and she later committed suicide. Evelyn could just imagine the flashbacks the patient must have had, and that the patient must have felt like the future would turn out as bad as the past. Evelyn felt horrible, especially since she thought that better utilization review might have helped the evaluator to be more cognizant of the risks in the case.

Although it turned out the mother was calling mainly to tell what happened and not to sue, they all realized utilization review needed to be approached differently, and asked their medical director to lead a meeting to see if they could bring U.B. to understand where he was wrong and persuade him to adjust accordingly. Before the meeting, The Bear reviewed U.B.'s authorizations and seemed to pick up a pattern of overzealous denial. He also felt a pang of guilt as he wondered if he had given U.B. too much free rein.

A BRIEF HISTORY

Although the record of performance to date made it look simpler to fire U.B. (for circumventing the appeal process, if nothing else), The Bear agreed that it would be worthwhile to try to put utilization review into a different perspective for U.B. and to salvage him for The Ethical Way if at all possible. He felt that U.B. was overemphasizing cost savings and putting patients at risk, possibly to please their chief financial officer, Buddy Richman. Realizing that U.B. was following common review practice and perhaps still had the potential to be effective and constructive on the job, he wanted U.B. to see how utilization review had gone from a welcome new process in the mental health professions to a cause of enormous controversy and ethical concerns.

So he gave a short history, and also suggested that U.B. later read the review articles by Jack Zusman, Steven Hoge, and Barry Blackwell. The Bear began with the way utilization review developed in mental health before it did in the rest of healthcare. It developed out of the concept and process of peer review, which started in the 1960s. In various kinds of institutions, psychiatrists would meet to chart review the treatment of other psychiatrists. Hospital utilization review started in the late 1960s and was associated with quality assurance. This was internal review, done by the hospitals themselves to provide an evaluation of the necessity, appropriateness, and efficiency of the hospital's services and facilities.

Review of cases by people outside the organization or clinician's workplace started a little later, in the 1970s, and began the process of utilization review on behalf of third-party payers. Provided by the American Psychiatric Association to the insurers of military personnel (CHAMPUS), this development highlighted many of the ethical issues that have subsequently developed. At that time CHAMPUS was concerned with abuse of psychiatric benefits, especially fraudulent claims and unnecessarily expensive treatment, both of which threatened to either bankrupt the program or drastically reduce mental health benefits. While there was some early dissent from colleagues—some of whom would call a reviewer a Judas goat—at its best it was thought to offer respected collegial feedback that would reinforce professional ego ideals.

The success of the reviews done by the American Psychiatric Association led to widespread use by insurers to approve payment for all kinds of healthcare. From being used by less than 10 percent of insurance plans in 1980, by 1990 some kind of utilization review was a feature of over 90 percent of health insurance plans. However, it is now perhaps ironic that the American Psychiatric Association (which has stopped doing utilization review) and other mental health organizations and numerous clinicians have come to feel that utilization review has become abusive in itself. Instead of the original goals of improving quality and saving money, there is concern that the only goal has come to be to save money.

"Do you think that goal fits you, U.B.?" The Bear growled.

Ready to fight back, U.B. thought better of it and replied, "Perhaps."

"Very well. Let me go on," The Bear snarled. Evelyn and Adam continued to sit and listen.

Utilization Review Today

Barry went on to explain that while many kinds of organizations and individuals can provide utilization review services, managed care companies have made it become a major tool for reviewing the so-called medical necessity of treatment. While at first emphasizing inpatient care, they now apply it to outpatient treatment also. Generally, there are no specific requirements, laws, or licensing agencies controlling who does reviews, so reviewers can be employed or contracted secretaries, nurses, social workers, psychologists, or psychiatrists.

"Even people like you, U.B.," The Bear snapped.

Usually, the review is done by phone, locally or from a national office, when treatment is about to begin or soon after. Reviews can be done at any frequency. Criteria for what is defined as medical necessity for the varieties of inpatient, day, and outpatient treatments are often deemed proprietary and not shared by managed care companies. The companies emphasize that their authorization is only for payment, but that the clinician can still see the patient and possibly work out other payment mechanisms if payment is not authorized. There is usually an appeals process available within the company, although recently Blue Cross/Blue Shield of Virginia had an appeal approval rate of less than 5 percent, and this probably isn't unusual. It may seem hypocritical for psychiatrists to complain about utilization review, for both business- and physician-controlled companies will usually reduce utilization. Usually, a written treatment plan is required, and sometimes records are requested and patients can be talked to directly.

"This is starting to sound a lot more like me," U.B. said more assertively.

"Wait before you feel too good about that," The Bear cautioned with a wave of his hand.

U.B., feeling a little less intimidated, fought back. He emphasized that the general results of utilization review seem clear for cost savings. Frequency and length of inpatient hospitalizations have dropped dramatically across the country. Brief or intermittent psychotherapy, provided mainly by nonpsychiatrists, is the norm and psychoanalysis or intensive long-term psychotherapy is rarely authorized. Psychiatrists are generally authorized only for hospitalization treatment, evaluation of complex cases, and fifteen-minute med checks. Managed care companies state that the cost savings are associated with more appropriate treatment by better clinicians. At its best, review can be an expert second opinion for everyone.

The Bear stood up and growled out, "Clinicians who work independently tend to see it differently. Clinicians will often claim that appropriate treatment is being denied, and that they are forced either to forgo usual reimbursement or provide treatment they feel is inadequate. Calling a utilization reviewer through an 800 number can often seem like calling 1–800–NO-YOU-CAN'T. Patients can come to feel confused as to who is responsible for what, and wonder what kind of insurance they have. Since each of the participants in this utilization review process is encountering different aspects of a general ethical challenge, that is, can utilization review provide more cost-effective treatment, let's now examine the different ethical angles separately. Maybe then you'll get what I'm trying to get at."

"Maybe," replied U.B. "But to me, the most similar medical activity to utilization review may be forensic evaluation. To put together a forensic evaluation of a defendant, so-called experts review clinical information very similar to what utilization reviewers get. The difference is, with utilization review, there's currently no judge or jury to provide an independent conclusion. But in all kinds of nonmedical fields, ranging from teachers to high-priced entertainers, there is review of performance, often with financial repercussions. Sometimes the reviews are done by those without the credentials of those being reviewed, such as a drama critic reviewing a play. So how can you judge what I've done?"

"I'm your boss, that's how, and you're working for a managed care company that is trying to pay special attention to ethics." Adam and Evelyn nodded vigorously with approval.

"I know that," responded U.B. "So what did I do wrong?"

Sensing U.B. still wasn't getting it, The Bear decided to attack U.B.'s emotions. "Don't you feel bad that our patient committed suicide? We want appropriate utilization review to include empathy for the business, the clinician, *and* the patient. Always think for a moment how you'd feel if one of your loved ones' treatment was being reviewed."

Now Evelyn and Adam appeared more sad.

"The Ethical Way wants to do everything it can to avoid the suicide way—or other bad outcomes for patients," Evelyn emphasized.

"Even if it costs us more money," Adam added.

The Utilization Reviewer

"You know," The Bear continued, "the people who have been doing basic utilization review have in essence been working in uncharted ethical territory. No special licensing or standardized training has existed, professional ethical codes have never addressed such an activity, and there's no published literature analyzing the comparative clinical outcomes of utilization review decisions. Strong rumors have circulated that companies set quotas or rewards for denial of claims, with threat of job loss for those who protest. It should be expected, then, that at least some utilization reviewers would be doing some ethical soul-searching, like you should be doing.

"Over the last ten years, two published accounts by people who worked as reviewers describe some of the ethical struggles. You should read these reports religiously, U.B., but let me summarize them now.

Even the titles, as similar as they are, imply some of the changes in being a reviewer over this decade. In 1986, the title includes the 'reflections' of a 'peer reviewer.' In 1996, we have the 'confessions' of a 'concurrent reviewer.' So, from the scholarly ruminations of a reviewer reviewing other peers, we have come to the soul-searching, guilt-considered confessions of reviewers who may or may not be reviewing peers.

"In 1986, Richard Parlour, a psychiatrist, described the peer review experience he shared with other reviewers as part of the CHAMPUS peer review process. Approximately 6 percent of cases were referred for peer review, while the rest were automatically authorized. The criteria used to assign cases for peer review in the early 1980s were pretty arbitrary: inpatient psychiatric stay of over sixty days, inpatient alcoholism stay of over twenty-one days, or over sixty outpatient visits. Exceptions could be made for earlier review. Generally, CHAMPUS followed the peer-review recommendations (by three different independent psychiatrists), which in one report, broke down to 55 percent full approval, 24 percent partial approval, 19 percent denial, and 20 percent voluntary termination by the treating clinicians.

"The reflections in the article emphasized some of the problematic treatments reviewed, including:

"*Sketchy listing of treatment modalities* without accompanying documentation that they were actually used in the referenced case.

"*Filing of claims for higher reimbursable services,* such as claiming residential as hospital, without any real change in treatment provided.

"*Misuse of inpatient services,* such as a child hospitalized for eighty-one days in an adult hospital for a simple school phobia or a hyperactive child hospitalized for four hundred days without a trial of either methylphenidate or antipsychotic medication.

"*Questionable outpatient psychotherapy,* such as ineffective therapy over six months to six years without consultation or trying alternative approaches, and psychotherapy justified only as a 'personal growth experience.'

"*Medication questions,* such as multiple cases where potentially addicting benzodiazepines were prescribed for substance abusers, or inadequate trials of appropriate medication.

"Parlour did not seem to describe much anguish in making recommendations, though there was some concern about how information was shared between the insurers and clinicians. He wondered, for instance, how well policy limits were conveyed and understood by clinicians. He concluded that cost-effectiveness was a legitimate requirement for reimbursement, including that less expensive modalities, such as medication, should often be tried before long-term psychotherapy, and that the CHAMPUS checkpoints were much too long.

"It's interesting, in view of where peer review is today, to note that although Parlour felt the eventual impact of peer review was hard to predict, he described the ethical dilemma of how to balance or weigh possible adverse effects versus possible benefits of peer review. For instance, he wondered whether such adverse effects as the increased expense or more defensive clinical practice would be worth more efficient use of resources and better identification of the most effective treatments."

U.B. seemed interested in these personal histories of utilization reviewers. "Go on, please."

Barry could hardly conceal his pleasure at hearing the word "please" from U.B. He doubted that U.B. ever used that word during his reviewing process. "Thank you," he responded. Then he continued in a more relaxed manner.

"By ten years later, peer review had evolved into utilization review, but many of the ethical questions remained. Paul Mohl—the author of the other article you should read—is an academic psychiatrist in charge of training new psychiatrists, and he also spent two years as an external reviewer for two managed care companies. By his time, guidelines for various intensities of treatment were further along. The criteria were often not deemed confidential and reviewers were apparently encouraged to discuss them with the clinicians.

"Mohl, too, encountered numerous examples of problematic treatment. In many cases, the clinician seemed to have little knowledge of the individual patient, and instead provided cookbook or canned treatments, such as twenty-eight-day inpatient programs for all substance abusers. Basic psychiatric skills, such as a good mental status examination, were absent. Depressed, suicidal patients could be hospitalized for a week without the initiation of antidepressants. Often, more convenient hospitalization was desired instead of extra outpatient work. Instead of whether sixty days was too long for hospitalization, now there were questions of whether eight hours a day of day treatment was better than four hours a day. Information was often missing and could even be contradictory or misleading."

"So that doesn't sound too different from the garbage I've been dealing with," U.B. commented.

"So far, but let me go on. Though Mohl also concludes that accountability must be externally applied to aspects of behavioral healthcare, his confessions reveal more personal moral struggles and system ethical dilemmas. He wonders whether he 'was being seduced or educated.' He 'was horrified' when told he was an extreme outlier in that he certified approval of treatment more often than other reviewers. He voiced uncertainty about the standard of care for difficult borderline patients. He found it hard to maintain a fluid balance in relating to the company, patients, and fellow psychiatrists. He came to conclude that some managed care companies seemed concerned only with saving money, while others tried to balance costs and quality. He recognized that the employer payers were both concerned about spending too much money on mental healthcare and angry whenever care was denied to one of their employees.

"One overall ethical concern seemed to be whether authorization for payment was indirectly coercing clinicians into certain practice patterns, and even reviewers into certain review patterns. Another ethical concern was whether managed care was on a slippery slope to certifying less care in the service of more profits. Though remaining ambivalent about the review process, he decided to stay involved and hoped that since utilization review was going to remain, that more good than bad would come from the process."

"I think I see what you mean," U.B. responded in a much humbled way.

"Perhaps," said The Bear.

"Dr. Mohl looks like a good model for utilization review," Evelyn added.

"Is he available?" Adam asked jokingly.

Understanding the Clinician's Perspective

"U.B., as you undoubtedly know," Barry began again, "utilization review has not been particularly popular among the clinicians whose treatment is being reviewed. Of course, some of that criticism may come from defensive clinicians who are overly confident about their own work, or who unconsciously need to deny their own limitations. Passive-aggressive behavior toward reviewers can then ensue.

"On the other hand, the sole reason can't be just that they don't like their treatment reviewed. After all, some clinicians will voluntarily ask for consultations for a second opinion in difficult cases. New clinicians will occasionally pay for supervision, recognizing that it can take years to become a seasoned clinician. Rather, as Glen Gabbard and many other clinicians claim, it is also for ethical and legal reasons that they are concerned about utilization review. They worry about things like these:

> "The process can take so long that the clinician has to treat before authorization is conveyed.

> "Patients harmed by premature hospital discharge usually sue the physician, not the insurer or reviewer—and if the insurer also gets sued, the physician is still deemed clinically responsible whether payment was authorized or not.

> "Adding a third party to the treatment can reinforce patient pathology, such as the splitting that occurs with borderline patients.

> "Pseudo improvement will seem to occur when patients and clinicians comply with external expectations."

Barry then asked U.B. to consider a case described by the psychiatrist Barry Blackwell. Dr. Blackwell was asked to do a consultation on a man who, following surgery, acted belligerent and confused. The patient belonged to an HMO that subcapitated its behavioral healthcare services to a managed care group outside the psychiatrist's hospital. Blackwell called the managed care company to request prior authorization, but the reviewer seemed to be asking questions that could only be answered if the consultation had already been conducted. The utilization reviewer then offered an outpatient appointment instead. After explaining that the patient was pulling out his tubes in an apparent delirium, the reviewer asked, "What is delirium?"

"My God, who would hire a reviewer like that?" exclaimed U.B.

"Somebody supposedly did, unless Blackwell was distorting the interaction for his own gain," replied Barry. "But I'm glad you're concerned about the qualifications for utilization reviewers. There are other times when utilization review can seem to be helpful to a clinician. Dr. Gabbard describes a utilization reviewer who acted like a collaborator with the treatment team, working toward a compromise that would balance cost concerns with clinical needs. In the case described, a thirty-three-year-old woman with refractory depression, serious suicide attempts, and twenty-seven brief hospitalizations was finally sent to a psychiatric hospital specializing in longer-term treatment. The reviewer attended a case conference two months later and actually authorized six more months of hospitalization. After six months, the reviewer suggested day treatment after a planned transition that allowed the patient to disengage from the hospital staff and start a new therapeutic alliance with the day treatment staff."

"Hmmm, that's quite generous. We couldn't do that, could we?" asked U.B.

"Why not? At least in special, rare cases," The Bear responded forcefully. He thought another perspective was still needed to do the trick for U.B.

The Patient's Point of View

"Patients are often surprised that utilization review even exists. A patient named Kate Walter, who recently wrote an op-ed piece called 'Give Me Therapy—Or Else' in the *New York Times*, described how surprised she was to find out that her therapist had a conversation with a representative from the managed care company, where the reviewer mentioned that her psychotherapy would no longer be covered unless it was based on medical necessity. With some irony, she wrote that it didn't pay to begin to get healthier; rather, she'd just about have to try to kill herself to remain in therapy. Not only was she displeased that someone else was finding out about her therapy, but that in turn the insurance company would not give her a definition of medical necessity."

"OK, OK, I'm getting the point," U.B. responded. "I don't need to hear about another patient suicide. I hear you already. In an attempt to save money, I've been denying some of the legitimate needs of patients and clinicians. Utilization review really can cause damage. That doesn't fit the ethical standards of my professional background."

Barry sensed that U. B. Wright would more readily live up to his name as a reviewer now. To be extra sure, he went over a few more cases.

Experimental Treatments

"U.B., a not too uncommon ethical consideration in utilization review is whether or not to cover so-called experimental or investigative treatments, especially if standard treatment has been unsuccessful. Things move so fast, sometimes the requested treatment wasn't known about at the time of the original policy or contract. In general medicine, this often comes up over requests for bone marrow transplants for cancer or new medications for AIDS. In behavioral healthcare, such considerations can arise in a case like this one:

"This case came up to the managed care company medical director for review in 1994 on an appeal by the patient's new therapist to provide EMDR—that's Eye Movement Desensitization and Reprocessing—therapy under her insurance coverage. The first level of review was done by the company utilization review nurse. The case had not been reviewed previously as the patient had recently obtained new insurance.

"The new therapist had filled out the standard treatment plan form asking to provide EMDR. The utilization review nurse asked for a case summary because this was an unusual request.

"The patient was a forty-three-year-old woman who was hospitalized four years prior, apparently for depression precipitated by fears of her parents' dying. She then continued in biweekly psychotherapy with unknown medication. Sometime over the four years she also suffered a job loss and also started to recall some prior trauma, perhaps during childhood. She apparently stopped taking medication earlier this year due to ongoing side effects. The treating psychiatrist then referred the patient to see the new therapist to do EMDR in addition to continuing her therapy and medication.

"The utilization review nurse then consulted with colleagues and a company psychiatrist consultant. They concluded that although there have been reported successes, especially with remnants of prior trauma, EMDR was still an unproven medical treatment requiring further research. It also seemed that in this case it was unclear whether more standard treatment had been unsuccessful or not. Although the information on prior treatment was spotty, especially regarding medication, prior psychotherapy seemed to have been of some help. These conclusions were conveyed to the new therapist, with the added possibility that the therapist could send additional information to support her request.

"What was returned was a written consultation from another psychologist who worked at the institution where the new therapist worked. Here's a copy." They all gathered round to read.

To Whom It May Concern:
I have been requested to comment on the claim that Eye Movement Desensitization and Reprocessing (EMDR) is an experimental psychotherapeutic procedure. At this point in its use, I strongly believe it should be considered the treatment of choice for the treatment of traumatic memories, rather than an experimental method. There are several reasons for this position:

1. There are more controlled studies supporting the effectiveness and efficiency of EMDR in treating the symptoms of PTSD than any other psychotherapeutic method. In addition, there is an extensive list of case reports pointing toward the effectiveness of EMDR. References are attached, as are several other studies that relate to this subject.

2. EMDR is widely used in the treatment of PTSD. At this time over 7,000 licensed mental health professionals have been trained in the use of EMDR. The attached survey of EMDR practitioners reports on the use of the method by the first 1,400 clinicians trained in it. As can be seen, they represent a wide cross-section of the mental health profession, and report positive results. Over thirty Veterans Administration Medical Centers have staff members who have been trained. In many of these medical centers EMDR is the PTSD treatment of choice by appropriately trained clinicians.

3. Of the many clinical settings where EMDR is in use, I know of none that require written consent for the use of EMDR. If EMDR was considered an experimental method, these facilities would be required to use such consent.

4. Some commentators of EMDR claim that its effectiveness can be completely explained by its similarity to the widely accepted behavioral principle of exposure. Though there are many reasons to doubt this opinion it is acknowledged that EMDR contains enough elements in common with other behavior techniques to be considered a cognitive behavioral therapy.

"The company medical director, who was not particularly familiar with EMDR, reviewed this letter and the accompanying attachments and concluded that the material did not support that EMDR was more than an experimental procedure, to wit: First, none of the material included a controlled, published study supporting EMDR's efficacy in a refereed, well-established journal. Second, while numerous clinicians and patients touted the effectiveness of EMDR, there were also numerous cases where EMDR did not seem effective or lost its effectiveness over time. In addition, the medical director concluded, he wasn't yet sure that this patient had actually suffered a prior trauma in the first place." Barry dropped out of lecture mode and turned to his unfortunate utilization reviewer. "So, U.B., do you agree so far, and what would be your final recommendation?"

"I would be comfortable in writing the following," U.B. replied after some thought. "While EMDR does seem to be a promising technique, it is still too early to consider it a medically established treatment. In this case, it is also unclear whether more standard treatment had been successful or not. If the patient still desired EMDR, that should be considered experimental and the patient could make her own independent financial arrangements."

"Good response," replied Barry. "As you know, the procedure I described for this case is not necessarily a standard utilization review process. Some managed care companies may have done less processing, a few perhaps more. Probably most would deny EMDR, but perhaps not all. Regardless of such variations, some generic ethical issues from the companies' standpoint exist, and I wonder how you would answer some ethical questions:

> *"Should unproven techniques be authorized on a case-by-case basis rather than denied under a blanket policy against so-called experimental treatments?"*

"I'd say you need a general policy or guideline," U.B. replied. "You could allow for exceptions, though, perhaps decided by an internal ethics committee or external ethics review board."

"I'd agree," said Barry, "and maybe have the internal committee as a first appeal, then the external board as the last step, given that patients could still pursue their own legal means. Next:

> *"Was having all the utilization review done internally and paid by the company a biased process supporting denial of cost-effective treatment?"*

"I wouldn't even have questioned whether our process was biased or not previously," U.B. replied, "but it sure has that potential."

"Precisely," said Barry. "That's why we always have to keep in mind the perspective and needs of the clinician and patient. If one of the goals of the company is to save money, and the reviewer doesn't have personal responsibility for the well-being of the patient, the review process can easily become stingy with authorizing and recommending necessary treatment. So:

> *"Was the company putting itself at more financial risk and the patient at more clinical risk by denying a treatment that might prevent the future need for hospitalization?"*

"Or worse maybe," answered U.B. "Not only would hospitalization be a risk, but maybe even suicide."

Barry began to wonder if U.B. was going overboard with empathy. "Well, as long as we got the patient to appropriate treatment, she should do all right. Next:

> *"Since EMDR was not even practiced at the time of the original contract with the payer, was the managed care company obligated to discuss this new treatment possibility with representatives from the payer?"*

"Yes," U.B. replied, "I'd say we need ongoing communications that would process new issues between contracts."

"Agreed," said Barry. "We need adjustments since new information might indicate a changed ethical decision."

Supporting Good Treatment

"U.B., you know that although utilization review has often focused on what treatment seems to be unnecessary or inappropriate, it can have another role. It also has the potential to reinforce what appears to be excellent treatment and even advocate for additional treatment. See what you think of this case:

The forty-year-old patient had used nineteen of her twenty authorized sessions. Almost a year before, she had an authorized psychiatric hospitalization following a suicide attempt—she'd been in an apparent dissociated state, and had a history of addictive behavior involving alcohol, food, and sex. There appeared to be a reliable history of extensive childhood sexual and psychological abuse. Outpatient therapy with another clinician before the hospitalization was not helpful. After some twice-weekly then weekly therapy, the patient was alcohol free, in better control of eating, and with less dissociation. However, her shame was still strong and she was considering divorcing her husband. She did not want to try medication or self-help groups.

"So what would your recommendation be in this case?"

"I would make the following conclusions," U.B. replied. "The patient seems to be following an expected course of successful psychotherapy for a posttraumatic or related disorder. While medication is worth considering, it often is not helpful in such conditions. Self-help groups may be helpful, but are not essential. Since a new benefit year is beginning and that allows up to twenty therapy sessions while the therapist is requesting only twelve, I would thank the therapist and authorize at least the twelve additional sessions."

"You'd actually offer the potential for more sessions than the therapist asked for?"

"Well, I hedged by saying 'at least,' but I can see there could be cases where it would be appropriate to tell the clinician to do more."

"Well, I'm glad we're being sensitive to the devastating aftermath of sexual trauma and abuse on women," Evelyn commented. "What sort of treatment is appropriate in such cases has been controversial in behavioral healthcare generally, but especially in managed care with its cost emphasis. Do you try to patch things up, or do you try for more substantial change? Do you try new faddish treatments or not?"

"Thanks for that perspective, Evelyn," replied Adam. "I was beginning to wonder why all these cases were starting to sound a little alike."

"Yes, mainly two men talking about issues concerning abused women," Evelyn responded with a little irritation. "And aren't most managed care companies run by men?"

"Well, this last case is a male—a thirteen-year-old with frequent behavioral problems, including substance abuse, running away, and school expulsion. He had three therapists and had been in several shelters. The parents were divorced. After two weeks of inpatient treatment, the attending psychiatrist recommended sixty to ninety days of residential treatment due to the prior unsuccessful outpatient attempts and family conflicts," Barry went on.

"The original utilization reviewers (a social worker and a psychiatrist) felt that medical necessity was met for a residential facility, but found out that this was not a covered benefit. They tried to make a case for approval of this alternative service to the payer employer. They provided the following financial information. 'The treatment program's standard cost is $240 discounted at 20 percent for a rate of $192 for a total cost of ninety times $192, or $17,280. David's acute inpatient stay has cost $335 per day for fifteen days, for a total cost of $5,025. The combined cost of both programs would be $22,640.' They also noted that if inpatient care had to be continued, the eventual cost would likely be higher.

"The employer company representative then made the final determination, writing, 'The outpatient benefit is $3,000 per person per calendar year. We are in violation of ERISA if we increase that amount selectively. I cannot make a decision in favor of the child. Perhaps the family can pursue community resources to get help for all family members. Each person requesting an exception has an earnest plea for help, but we are required to administer benefits based on published documented provisions, and to treat all employees the same. Sorry, I cannot grant this request.'"

"Too bad," responded U.B. "That alternative treatment plan seemed appropriate."

"Right," replied Barry. "So, unfortunately, despite the support of the reviewers and the managed care company, the employer denied the request for special services. Further processing of the issues in this case, however, led to residential care becoming a new possible written benefit as an alternative to hospitalization."

"Well, I think you've got it now, U.B.," Barry continued after a pause. "Let's work together more closely so we can follow The Ethical Way of doing utilization review."

"And we'll work closer with you, Barry, since we're all in this together," Evelyn added.

STANDARDS

"An excellent—albeit long—meeting," concluded Adam. "I wonder if we can produce some written standards related to our discussion. In my software company, we always had written standards."

"Yes, I'm sure we can," Barry responded, "although it's hard for me to equate us with software. Just as we went through the relevant parties in discussing utilization review ethical challenges, let's do the same for possible solutions. Maybe we can alternate. I'll go first and cover the payers."

Payers

"Payers should make sure utilization review is used as much to improve treatment as to save money. What would you recommend for managed care companies, U.B.?"

Managed Care Companies

"Managed care companies should hire competent reviewers who will only review areas of care within their own clinical competence, and the company should set up an appeals process that will reduce conflict of interest as much as possible. The company should belong to, and accept the standards of, the National Utilization Review Accreditation Commission, as long as that seems to be an unbiased organization.

"What constitutes investigation or experimental treatment should be clearly defined, and not too rigidly to exclude commonly accepted traditional treatments that may not yet have been subject to extensive research.

"Would you like to cover utilization review, Barry, as it may be an ethical conflict of interest to me to do so?" continued U.B. with a smile.

"Yes, I'd be glad to," Barry replied, "especially since I have so many recommended solutions."

Utilization Reviews

"Reviewers should have as their ultimate goal to provide a helpful second opinion within the financial constraints of the contract.

"Here I suggest we adopt some of the recommendations of Stephen Green:

"The reviewers should try to develop a review alliance with the clinician akin to a psychotherapy therapeutic alliance.

"The reviewer must be able to demonstrate expertise without condescending to the clinician.

"The reviewer must monitor such countertransference potential as overidentification, narcissism, and competition.

"The reviewer should be comfortable with setting appropriate limits.

"The reviewer should sustain primary ethical responsibility to the profession.

"In addition to those of Dr. Green, I would add:

"Be careful of unnecessary destruction of patient care.

"The threat of using the power to withhold payment may be helpful enough in reducing a lot of unnecessary care.

"An ethical reviewer or review process will at least at times recommend more treatment rather than less."

"What would you now recommend for clinicians, U.B.?"

Clinicians

"This interaction has really gotten me more in touch with my prior career as a clinical psychologist," U.B. replied, "and if I were doing that again, here is what I would recommend for clinicians:

"Accept the possibility that utilization review could be helpful for the care of a patient, and guard against inappropriate passive-aggressive behavior.

"Discuss the process with patients at the first visit as part of regular informed consent.

"Make sure that appropriate consent for exchange of information gets signed.

"Follow appropriate legal guidelines such as in the case of substance abuse treatment in a facility receiving federal funds.

"Make sure that the reviewer is who he says he is by calling the company he says he is from to check that it's true.

"Only reveal information relevant to the utilization review decision.

"Keep careful records of both the clinical and utilization review process.

"Appeal if you disagree with the reviewer.

"Be your own utilization reviewer, trying to guide treatment planning in cost-effective ways and knowing of any available relevant research and literature that will objectively support your intervention strategy.

"That's all I've got for now. What's next, Barry?" asked U.B.

The Law

"Well, we haven't discussed legal responses to utilization review too much," Barry responded after a pause, "but lawsuits and state regulations are starting. I would hope that legal consideration of the utilization review process will continue to determine where the clinician's responsibility ends and the managed care company's responsibility begins. So I would recommend that

> "The law and legislation needs to continue to grapple with how close utilization review is to the actual practice of medicine and to develop standards, licensing, and review processes accordingly.

> "State legislators should adopt a regulation that the utilization review process must conform to basic community standards, akin to the legal principle of community standards for mental health treatment, so that reasonable time needs to be spent doing the reviews and necessary records reviewed.

> "As Steven Hoge, M.D., has discussed, we should reconsider the federal ERISA law, which preempts many plans from following healthcare standards while instead allowing utilization review decisions to be based on business."

Although Barry was quite pleased with U.B.'s development, and felt that good review of treatment was ethically justified for the best interests of patients as well as costs, he also felt that utilization review in this form would run its course. In its present form, it was still too subjective or idiosyncratic due to the individual knowledge of the reviewers. If guidelines were followed too rigidly, individual variation would be neglected. In the future, networks of clinicians would likely become more cost-effective in their approach and be supplemented by sophisticated technological treatment monitoring.

BUSINESS VERSUS BEHAVIORAL HEALTHCARE ETHICS SCORECARD

Evelyn and Adam were quite pleased with these standards. The standards offered some solutions to the ethical challenges of the utilization review concept.

If this kind of utilization review had been available at the time, they thought the inpatient scandals of the early 1990s—which followed the discovery that hospital patients were being captured and kept overly long—might have been avoided. On the other hand, they didn't want to see new scandals from too little treatment. Their own patient suicide might have been averted. The current ethical challenge was for utilization review to operate in a manner that will help to produce the most cost-effective quality treatment possible. But until that day arrived—for better or worse—the utilization review game would continue. So Adam suggested yet another exhibition game with the following rules:

- *Both healthcare and business ethics win* if utilization review both reduces unnecessary care and increases necessary care, without adversely affecting the patient-clinician relationship.

- *Business ethics win but healthcare ethics lose* if utilization review indiscriminately reduces all treatment and compromises helpful patient-clinician alliances.

- *Healthcare ethics win but business ethics lose* if good treatment is always approved but behavioral healthcare costs rise dramatically.

- *Both sides lose* if related social costs such as lowered work productivity and medical costs such as psychosomatic symptoms develop because behavioral healthcare coverage is even further reduced due to an inability of mental health clinicians to work out a helpful monitoring system of checks and balances.

Evelyn and Adam were now becoming secure that their managed care company was on sound business and ethical healthcare footing. But with all the changes in the field, including mergers, new opportunities, and new competition, they thought they needed to develop a three-year plan that would keep them on the ethical way for the twenty-first century.

CHAPTER TEN

Future Challenges

B y now, Evelyn Bloom and Adam Wilder, co-owners of The Ethical Way, felt that their managed behavioral healthcare company was getting off to a reasonable start. Clinically, no disasters had occurred and outcome studies were looking positive. Financially, things were tight, but at least they weren't losing money.

Although they had always intended to do things "the ethical way," they were a little surprised at how many ethical issues and challenges there were, once you tried to pay attention to them. As their one-year anniversary approached, they reminisced about their struggles to

- Balance business ethics with healthcare ethics.

- Try to infuse ethical principles throughout the company.

- Find the most cost-effective gatekeeping process.

- Provide adequate informed consent to patients and providers.

- Maintain adequate confidentiality.

- Have financial influences motivate neither to undertreat nor to overtreat.

• Provide the best treatment possible under the financial and societal parameters of their contracts.

• Use utilization review for a valuable second opinion rather than for an excuse to deny treatment.

So, after a long day at the office, Evelyn asked Adam where he thought they were at.

"Do you mean personally?" Adam said smilingly.

"No, I mean the company," Evelyn replied, blushing. "I mean, we've done pretty well in meeting our ethical challenges, we've both won or tied in our ethical exhibition games, and we've meshed our value systems adequately. But managed care is changing so rapidly and we still haven't solved our ethical challenges, maybe we need to do some more planning."

"I'm glad you feel we've meshed well," Adam responded. "I certainly agree. And perhaps ethical challenges are never resolved. But you're right, managed care continues to develop quickly. Hey, how about bringing all of our employees together for a one-year anniversary 'State of The Ethical Way' address? We could each comment on our particular area of focus, me more on business ethics and you more on behavioral healthcare ethics."

"A great idea," Evelyn responded. "And let's also invite our consultants who have been so helpful."

Two weeks later, they rented a meeting room at a hotel to make their presentation. Adam spoke first.

"Welcome, everybody. And thanks for all you've done to help our company take the ethical way. I'm sure that it has been tempting to take other paths. But we've not only survived, I believe we've shown that it is possible for managed behavioral healthcare to solve its ethical challenges. Evelyn and I will share some of the ways we think we've met the challenges successfully, then we'll turn toward the future.

"First of all, we were determined to join the traditions of behavioral healthcare ethical principles and the best of business ethics. To do so, we reviewed the histories of each tradition to help us avoid repeating old mistakes. Then we developed a simple mission statement, 'the ethical way is the best possible joining of behavioral healthcare and business ethics,' which you're probably all sick of by now—we've been attaching that to virtually every communication, including your paycheck stubs."

There was some laughter and polite applause.

"Then we've tried to set up a system that would operationalize this mission statement. Though of course we've made some mistakes along the way, we've tried to hire people with the highest character like yourselves. We've used a top organizational consultant, Peter Woods, who is here with us. And we've also used an ethics consultant, Sun-Yu Moon, who is also here. That way we wouldn't be blinded by our own biases. We've made initial steps to set up a formal ethics committee that would meet monthly and as needed to review ethical challenges. Though we've included consumers, family members, and clinicians in our administrative conferences, we're about to set up an advisory board consisting of representatives of these constituencies as well as a governmental representative. We've been able to form a mutually satisfying educational and research venture with a local academic center.

"I hope we're at least at stage four of the five stages that Linda Starke discusses about corporate moral development. Stage four fits the emergent ethical corporation, where the company balances societal ethical concerns and the profit motive, including the admission of ethical mistakes. Do you agree?"

Adam noted rows of affirmative nods and even thought he heard a faint cheer sounding something like "Hey, hey, it's The Ethical Way!" Buoyed by the response, he continued.

"Finances have been the greatest temptation. We could have taken the financial way by denying services or shortchanging clinicians to make short-term high profits. But that would not have been The Ethical Way. We've started slow and within our means to maintain financial viability. We've turned down contracts that appeared to have inadequate capitation. And I'm most pleased to allay any rumors that we will be bought out by one of the huge national companies. No, we're in it for the long haul, at least until managed care or some other way of doing things leads to widespread high-quality, cost-effective behavioral healthcare. We're also almost ready to begin a profit-sharing process with all of you."

Adam stopped for stronger clapping, and the cheer became clearer, "Hey, hey, it's The Ethical Way."

"Finally, before I stop, let me say that it looks like our outcome studies are indicating that we can produce a successful one-tier system of care for patients of varying sociocultural backgrounds. With our Medicaid contract in particular, I believe we're showing that managed care principles can be applied to that group. And we continue to advocate wherever we can in political circles for parity for behavioral healthcare so that better financial coverage is available."

"Now let me turn this address over to my partner, Evelyn Bloom, M.D., who has been watching over the clinical side of our operation, which is why we're in business in the first place. Though second on the agenda today, patient care should still be first on our minds. Evelyn."

Even stronger clapping ensued for Evelyn.

"Thank you, Adam, and thanks to all of you. There's much to be proud of from the clinical side, so let me try to summarize the ethical challenges we faced. The first challenge was how to set up a gatekeeping process so that patients could be evaluated quickly and well so they would see the most appropriate clinician. Although we're still not sure, and our research comparison of various options is still proceeding, it appears that using master's level mental health clinicians who are warm, active, and knowledgeable works best, as long as psychiatrists are available for assessment of complex cases and later review of the written summaries to make sure something important wasn't missed. Using family practitioners is not the way to go, at least for now.

"We've upgraded our feeble original policies on informed consent, so that patients receive any relevant information on our company and how it affects their treatment, including the name of their utilization reviewer. There are no gag rules for clinicians. In fact, we are considering bonuses for those clinicians who do best on patient satisfaction surveys for providing information.

"After a major breach of confidentiality, we've tightened protection for the patient. Though we're using a sophisticated new management information system, we've put in enough passwords and checks to keep information more confidential than I think it was with written records.

"Now to treatment, the key to whatever success we've achieved. We've developed a multidisciplinary clinical network of community providers as well as employing the multidisciplinary staff of a community mental health center. The center staff is here, and we should especially applaud their efforts. They've accepted the need to consider costs in the provision of high-quality care. We've emphasized that treatment should be based on clinical research, when available, and not just on clinician or patient preference or experience. We've contracted with staff with such specialized skills as cross-cultural competence, child expertise, geriatric experience, dual-diagnosis, the creative arts, and skills with the aftermath of trauma. And we even pay these people more! Whenever possible, clinicians provide continuity of care across services.

"We've used utilization review so that only medically necessary treatment would be authorized. Though perhaps overzealous at first in denials—" she glanced with a smile toward U.B., "I think our utilization review has evolved into a valued second opinion. For appeals, to avoid conflict of interest, we've begun to experiment with the use of external reviewers, independent of our company. I think soon we will need less and less utilization review as our system incorporates the treatment philosophy of The Ethical Way. Outcome studies will show if this is the right way.

"Finally, I feel we're contributing to the future by educating students in the managed care way.

"Thanks to all of you. You're The Ethical Way."

Now the applause swelled and Evelyn, too, thought she heard the cheer, "Hey, hey, it's The Ethical Way."

"Thanks, Evelyn," Adam said as he joined her.

Later, after some good food and a little wine, some of the core administrative staff and consultants continued to discuss the future of The Ethical Way.

"Thanks for the encouraging summary and update," U.B. began. "I wonder if you could put our company in perspective and describe how you view managed behavioral healthcare nationally, especially from the ethical standpoint."

A NATIONAL PERSPECTIVE

"Well, I guess I can begin," Adam responded. "Nationally, there are megamergers of the biggest for-profit companies, more provider-owned new companies, and new contract opportunities, especially in Medicaid and Medicare. With these changes, we'll probably only have more ethical issues. I wonder if you could elaborate, Peter, as you've been so helpful to us as an organizational consultant."

Peter said that it was obvious that managed behavioral healthcare had been devoting the most attention to cost containment, and that at least up to now it appeared to have been successful to some degree. Entrepreneurial trials at company size, ownership, and operational strategies were still going on. Although there was a lot of rhetoric about attention to quality, that had just begun. While managed care had largely been a business development allowed—if not stimulated—

by government, now government—both state and national—was starting to take a greater role. Clinicians, also called providers, had become more and more outspoken on their opinions about managed care, and patients were now beginning to speak out and media coverage was increasing. "So, Sun-Yu, what do you think the ethical outcomes of these managed behavioral healthcare changes have been?"

Sun-Yu pondered for a while. "Although there is some literature out there to answer your question, it is scattered and limited. Let's see if we can pull it together, piece by piece, since there are so many ethical issues and challenges."

Costs

"As you indicated in your summary, Peter, cost has received the greatest attention in managed behavioral healthcare, so let's look first at the ethical outcomes here. The most ethical outcome is also the most simplistic, to wit:

> *"Managed behavioral healthcare has made costs an explicit healthcare ethical consideration."*

"Could you elaborate, Sun-Yu?" asked Peter. "Haven't costs always been a consideration?"

"Yes, costs have always been a consideration, but the differences in service were taken for granted by most. Different cost considerations existed in fee-for-service paid by the patient, indemnity insurance, and governmental plans. Mental healthcare was generally less well covered than other healthcare. Clinicians for the most part were able to influence their reimbursement, and, if anything, had a financial incentive to overtreat. Fraud by hospitals and clinicians is well known, up to 10 percent as reported by one Blue Cross company."

"Right," interjected Buddy from the audience, "and managed behavioral healthcare is changing all of that in a more businesslike way."

"Correct," replied Sun-Yu, "but whether the change is better or worse ethically is the question. For another change, we can note that

> *"Managed behavioral healthcare has apparently been paying less for behavioral healthcare than traditional indemnity insurance or other countries like Canada pay for the same service."*

"That's probably just cutting away the unnecessary fat," Buddy replied.

"Perhaps, but what's that cutting doing for all those people out there who need treatment? We know they're there, but they don't come in for one reason or another even if they have insurance, let alone that this country still has large numbers of people with no or limited insurance coverage. From an ethical standpoint, it seems to me that the country needs to find ways to bring into treatment those who need it, and managed care doesn't seem to have met that challenge at all," Sun-Yu responded.

"And the ethical irony with the uninsured, Sun-Yu, seems to be that they can end up in our community mental health system, funded by our governments, and sometimes receive better mental healthcare than people in the managed care or private sector," responded Evelyn.

"Correct again, but the plot thickens because now managed care is coming into the public sector," added Sun-Yu.

"And that will take care of some of the freeloaders and governmental bureaucracy," Buddy chimed in.

"Ah, but you lead into another ethical irony, another ethical behavioral issue:

"Where the money now goes in managed behavioral healthcare is different from where it used to go."

"If you mean that more money goes to profits and administrators, that's true," responded Buddy, "but that comes out of what we save the payers and is perfectly acceptable in business ethics."

"But is it acceptable in healthcare ethics?" Evelyn asked. "It would only be acceptable in healthcare ethics if it didn't worsen patient care in general."

"So we have another ethical cost consideration," Sun-Yu responded:

"Managed care financial operations tend to reward less treatment."

"But is that fine if that's adequate enough?" asked Buddy.

"But is it adequate?" Sam answered—like a good psychiatrist—with another question.

"Didn't Barry, our medical director, tell us that while research so far didn't show grossly poorer treatment results for managed care, that the jury was still out because the studies were so limited?" Adam pointed out.

"Unfortunately from healthcare ethical standpoint, that's correct," replied Sun-Yu. "Managed care has developed so fast, neglecting to study treatment effects along the way, that it is getting close to being too late for comparative studies of managed care versus traditional systems."

"Enough discussion on costs, I think," Adam interrupted. "We could go on and on, but are there other areas you have questions about?"

Treatment

"Sun-Yu, if we turn to the other part of managed care's typically stated goal of being cost-effective, we turn from costs to effective treatment. What ethical effects do you see here?" asked Evelyn.

"Another way of phrasing the question may be turning from the business ethics emphasis on costs to the healthcare ethics emphasis on treatment," added Adam.

"That is a good way to describe our main ethical pillars, Adam," replied Sun-Yu. "Just as with costs, it appears that with treatment managed behavioral healthcare has produced some clear ethical benefits along with possible ethical problems. The most positive ethical outcome to date, as with costs, is also quite simple, to wit:

> *"Managed behavioral healthcare has made treatment variations a primary healthcare ethical consideration."*

"But what do you mean, Sun-Yu?" asked Sam right away. "I mean, we've always had research examining new treatments, lots of supervision of students, and some peer review. Our most important ethical standard is the fiduciary one to put patients first."

"Ah yes, but all of that didn't help patients find an appropriate provider quickly, and didn't reduce unnecessary or inappropriate care or correct the social neglect of social variables in the biopsychosocial treatment model that most behavioral clinicians ascribe to."

"But what evidence is there that managed care has done better in that regard?" asked Stacy, the social worker. "Who has confirmed that managed care providers are better, that there aren't more subtle detriments to reducing treatment, and that the social component—if you mean money—isn't dominant now over biology and psychology in the treatment process?"

"Those are all good questions, Stacy," Sun-Yu responded. "That suggests another current ethical outcome that is similar to the problems managed care professes to address:

"Just as troubling as the wide variability in the quality of treatment by clinicians is the apparent wide variability in the quality of managed care companies."

"Yes!" cried out Seth, a psychologist at the mental health center. "So don't we need report cards on managed care companies just as much as we need report cards on clinicians?"

As Sun-Yu was about to agree, Adam broke in, "We're certainly agreeable to report cards on our company, provided they're done by an outside source without a conflict of interest."

"Just as should be done with report cards on clinicians like Stacy and me," Seth responded.

"Yes, and we already know that report cards have helped to improve treatment in medicine, so they should do the same in behavioral healthcare if well done," commented Sun-Yu.

"Do you think they'd do that by getting clinicians to follow common guidelines?" asked Seth. "And if so, where does that leave patient variation?"

"Good questions—pointing to another mixed ethical outcome so far," replied Sun-Yu.

"Managed behavioral healthcare has stimulated the production of many treatment guidelines, but the guidelines may differ, may be untested, and may not account for certain patient variations."

"Yes, those guidelines can be as much of a hindrance as help," Evelyn responded. "Just look at the medical guidelines that came out of some managed care companies for a twenty-four-hour hospital stay for vaginal births and a forty-eight-hour stay for cesareans. Sure, my own six-day stay was probably unnecessarily long and cesarean lengths of stay differed dramatically across the country, but the new guidelines seemed to cause enough rehospitalizations and deaths to produce lawsuits and some state legislation mandating longer stays."

"And all the while, physicians were getting sued for malpractice, while many managed care companies were able to claim exemption under ERISA," added Sam.

"Fortunately, it appears that the managed behavioral healthcare guidelines haven't produced as disastrous results, but we do have a lot of anecdotal reports of unnecessary suicides," added Evelyn.

"The trouble with anecdotal bad results is we don't know if such suicides were just as common before managed care, but didn't receive the same attention," commented Sun-Yu.

"And what about the other managed care effects on the treatment process," added Stacy, "like less informed consent, less confidentiality, less ethnic minority clinicians in networks, and more unqualified reviewers?"

"Also all good questions," answered Sun-Yu, "that I think are still unanswered. So we get

> *"When managed behavioral care alters traditional healthcare ethical principles like confidentiality, the burden of proof is on the new system to show that benefits outweigh the ethical changes."*

"The last ethical question I have for you on treatment, Sun-Yu," resumed Stacy, "is about the stewardship principle we keep hearing about, that clinicians have to keep societal needs in mind besides those of patients. Well, social workers have always kept society in mind, and codes of other disciplines at least mention societal needs, but where do we draw the line? After all, couldn't Nazi psychiatrists claim they were just following their societal goals when they helped kill off the mentally ill for the benefit of German society?"

"I agree that from a clinician's standpoint, considering societal needs as much as an individual patient's can be a slippery slope, so that the individual patient may still have to come first, but supplemented by more attention to cost-effectiveness. The problem could be stated like this:

> *"For an individual clinician with an individual patient, it is often not clear how to ethically balance the treatment needs of that patient with the needs of society."*

"What may help us with all of these ethical treatment dilemmas is more outcome studies," Adam suggested. "Maybe we're finally starting to look at quality for real after the industry has focused so much on cost and only gave lip service to quality. And the results of GTE's own internal company rankings are interesting, especially for those who hold high-flying healthcare stocks. Of the twenty-one managed care plans in the top 15 percent of quality, not one was a for-profit plan. Businesses are also coming to realize that just like clinicians, when managed care companies report on their own perceived quality, they are often inaccurate."

"Thanks for that promising report on payers' increasing concern with outcomes and quality," Sun-Yu commented.

Business Ethics

"Speaking about businesses, haven't both the payers and the managed care companies produced an enormous change in ethical priorities in managed behavioral healthcare?" Peter asked.

"Surely," answered Adam. "It reminds me some of the ethics in the software industry. The overriding ethic is to build a successful company, and successful in terms of profitable. Of course, we would always say that our innovations would help society by helping to make people's lives easier, but I don't believe the welfare of society was our main goal."

"So what you're saying is that perhaps business ethics have become as important as healthcare ethics in managed care, correct?" asked Peter.

"Yes, I'd even go so far as saying that we are in the process of the industrialization of health and behavioral healthcare," replied Adam. "We've got a product—medically necessary treatment; we've got the parts of the product—the type of treatment, the number of sessions, the length of stay; we've even got quality control—the selection of clinician workers and the utilization review of the workers."

"So I suppose the ongoing ethical question here has to do with whether business ethics are appropriate for healthcare," Peter responded. "It reminds me of the traditional separation of church and state in our country. In the past, we've had a strong degree of separation of business and healthcare. Were there sound ethical reasons to have had that separation? What do you think, Sun-Yu?"

"I think the essential ethical issue is whether pursuing business ethics compromises healthcare ethics in a way that is unacceptable to society, or in other words:

"Business ethics are producing a different behavioral healthcare product, but it is unclear as yet whether the product is better for society as a whole and adaptable enough for individual patient needs."

Governmental Ethics

"Speaking of society," Sun-Yu continued, "isn't our government supposed to represent the values of our people? So far it seems our government has more represented managed care businesses. We had Nixon's government, which helped pass laws to stimulate the growth of HMOs. Until recently, legislators and policymakers have allowed managed care companies to make their own decisions about the extent to which economic decisions should be incorporated into healthcare treatment decisions. One exception has been the state of Oregon, which developed a priority list of covered illnesses—in which behavioral problems fared well—through political, professional, and public input. Certainly, other countries have approached healthcare financing differently. We are the only country without a national health plan. Other countries seem to value the common good more than we do."

"Yet isn't even Canada now starting to turn more to managed care to manage its healthcare costs?" asked Evelyn.

"Correct, but maybe managed care principles will be applied differently there," suggested Sun-Yu. "Our government so far has focused on what is affordable rather than on what is good."

"Agreed," said Peter. "But maybe the government is having another chance now. Now that managed care is extending into Medicaid and Medicare, the states and the federal government have a new opportunity to shape and monitor how managed care functions. In Wisconsin's preliminary deliberations, I understand that the state is demanding that managed care delivery systems must result in three measurable outcomes: higher-quality care, better client outcomes, and the opportunity for savings to the state and counties."

"Sounds good," responded Sun-Yu with a note of skepticism. "At least there seem to be some new initiatives. And the federal Substance Abuse and Mental Health Services Administration (SAMHSA) established a position of director for a managed care initiative in 1995, with some initial projects centering on monitoring, developing standards, and supporting relevant research for managed behavioral healthcare networks."

"Maybe they should consider a goal like this ethical outcome," suggested Evelyn:

"Managed behavioral healthcare should help preserve life by reducing suicides, homicides, and self-destructive behavior; support liberty by allowing appropriate freedom of choice of clinicians by patients; and aid the pursuit of happiness by providing treatment that reduces depression and other psychological barriers to that pursuit."

A THREE-YEAR PLAN

"Well, we've had a nice review of the state of ethical outcomes in managed behavioral healthcare up to now both for us and nationally," Adam continued. "Some seem good, some questionable, and some just emerging. Are there any other questions or comments before we go home?"

Izzy, the student intern, raised his hand. "I must admit I've been much more impressed with your system than I thought I'd be. It's really broadened my perspective on ethical behavioral healthcare. I wonder where you feel you're headed in the next few years, especially since I may be looking for a job then!"

"Part of your question seems easier to answer than the other," Adam answered after a pause. "We do plan to be in existence for the next three years. So if you're finished by the year 2000 come and see me. We're planning on growing in a slow but sure ethical way.

"I sure hope we'll be able to reduce our administrative costs below 10 percent and closer to 5 percent. We also plan to have more students like you who can provide effective but low-cost treatment.

"The next population we hope to get a contract for is the Medicare population. I'm worried that group will be especially vulnerable to promises of more for less money. Moreover, the overlap of medical and behavioral healthcare problems that are so important in many of these patients calls for an integrated contract to cover both kinds of problems. Beyond that, I'm not sure. Are you, Evelyn?"

"No, managed care seems to be changing and growing so rapidly, it's hard to predict one year, let alone three years or five years."

"Agreed." Adam continued. "It seems like we will have to be ready to try to adapt to changes in the managed care environment around us, if it seems like the ethical way!"

"Perhaps we can at least let Izzy know what we hope the changes may be over the next three years," Evelyn suggested. "Sun-Yu, do you think you can start us off here?"

Government

"Fine," began Sun-Yu. "As I believe the great baseball player Yogi Berra once said, "If you don't know where you are going, you could end up somewhere else."

Even Adam had to laugh.

"It seems to me that the healthcare industry is just too complex and too vital to our nation for our government to stand on the sidelines. There seems to be so many ethically based things the government could do to help improve managed behavioral healthcare in the future, things I know The Ethical Way would like, including:

"The federal government must have an oversight role.

"The federal government should set budget guidelines for healthcare, with parity for behavioral healthcare.

"Federal legislation needs to regulate the playing field for developing managed care models, especially in the antitrust areas that limit the development of professionally led companies.

"The federal government should develop standards for essential behavioral healthcare services akin to what was done under community mental health services.

"The federal government should help the states by making sure they have adequate funding, clear mandates that are financially feasible, and the freedom to develop different managed care models.

"The state governments should slowly develop managed care programs with Medicaid populations, slowly enough to allow outcome comparisons with traditional systems.

"The state governments should require any managed care organization that contracts with the state for Medicaid patients to put aside at least 3 percent of any profits to a pool for medical education and research.

"All governments should monitor and punish fraud.

"Governments have an ethical responsibility to the underinsured and uncovered."

"Interesting recommendations, Sun-Yu," Peter responded. "I would certainly agree that our governments should have more of an oversight role. That seems like a different role from the one they had with the community mental health movement, when they funded, developed, and managed it directly."

"Correct," answered Sun-Yu. "The ethical problem with the government's role in community mental health was that its maintenance was dependent upon who was in power in Washington, leading to changed funding and guidelines to the extent that, just to survive, community mental health centers have gone off in many different directions other than their original intent."

"So what kind of oversight would you suggest, Sun-Yu?" Peter asked.

"It could take various forms. As the psychiatrist Peter Kramer has recommended, we could have an agency that monitors health insurance the way the FAA monitors aviation—so that we don't have crashes with no black box to indicate what went wrong."

"In principle that sounds like a good model," replied Evelyn, "but the mother in me needs to comment that the FAA hasn't stopped children from flying airplanes, one of which crashed recently."

"Thank you for that important example," Sun-Yu replied. "Until Jessica's tragic death, there wasn't much outcry by the aviation industry, the FAA, and the public about children piloting. If I can be immodest, another possibility for oversight might be a national bioethics commission or board, which would consist of representatives—without significant conflicts of interest—from relevant segments of life. In addition, akin to a personal financial advisor, each patient could have the potential availability of a managed care advisor to help understand benefits, amount of coverage, and options."

"I would support you on that," Peter responded. "How about budget guidelines and parity? Do you have numbers in mind?"

"Not really," replied Sun-Yu, "because it depends first of all what our other national priorities are. I mean, we could say healthcare should be 25 percent of our national GNP if other priorities lessen, or that behavioral healthcare should have more than parity because of the importance of mental well-being for the country. Then you have the whole question of what should be included in behavioral healthcare. Should there be an inclusion of some social services, which are so crucial for the seriously and chronically mentally ill? What about for child abuse wrap-around services, including such nontreatment services as child care, transportation, and housing? They've all shown their value in helping very troubled families. Preventive services geared to producing healthy families, less violence, and reduced substance abuse, while more costly at first, are likely to reduce medical and social costs in the long run."

"And, unfortunately, it looks like the maintenance or preventive part of health maintenance organizations has gone by the wayside in favor of company profits," added Peter. "It seems like in recommending more models for managed care, you're worried we haven't had enough variety yet, even with the multitude of different managed care plans."

"Yes, I'd at least like to see more clinician-owned systems, although so far it looks like when clinicians own managed care systems they run them just like entrepreneurs," Sun-Yu replied.

Too softly for anyone to hear, Evelyn muttered, "Sounds like identification with the aggressor to me."

Sun-Yu continued, "Another model would be to see if government-run systems, like community mental health centers, can adapt and compete with the new managed care systems for Medicaid contracts. We'll likely need some leading changes to help this along, such as a change in the ERISA law that protects self-insured companies from state healthcare regulations. Federal antitrust laws, which exempt insurance companies but not solo practitioners, also seem to need amending."

"As for essential services, would you suggest the government just recommend some of the traditional community mental health services—outpatient, inpatient, emergency, consultation and education—or go beyond them?" Evelyn asked.

"I'd at least like to see the services community mental health provided, especially the consultation and education to community services that are rarely done anymore, but that will depend on how much money is available," replied Sun-Yu.

"You also mentioned some of the things you think the state governments should ethically do, especially to go slowly, try to set up pilot trials, and set aside money for education and research," Peter went on. "The large numbers of mentally ill patients in some systems, 50,000 or more, seem like a potential gold mine for research."

"Yes, the states have a chance to slow down the managed care train and really reassess how well it delivers its product before there is no other way to do so," Sun-Yu replied.

"Though, of course, we don't want to slow managed care so much that its helpful experiments stop or the whole system crashes," cautioned Adam.

"Perhaps," replied Sun-Yu, "though certainly the government could decide that other systems, say, single payer or medical savings accounts, would serve the people better. Then, of course, along the way any form of government should be monitoring for fraud and abuse. The verified reports of some managed care company employees forging the names of Medicaid people to add to their numbers and breaking confidentiality to find out the names of healthy people are among the unethical and illegal practices the governments should watch closely. And what about the uninsured? Although coverage to some populations, like in Oregon, has expanded with managed care cost savings, the vast numbers of uninsured are still there. Moreover, as hospitals and clinicians see their reimbursement decreased, they seem less willing to offer free care. Is The Ethical Way or its clinicians offering any free care when coverage runs out, or even as a public service to those 40 million without any coverage at all?"

Evelyn and Adam were a bit taken back by this. They realized that as ethical as they tried to be they still didn't—or perhaps couldn't— go far enough and that some sort of government help or intervention was needed. They adjourned for the night and invited everyone to come by the office the next day for more discussion if they wanted to.

That night Evelyn had a nightmare about a patient tragedy—a psychiatric managed care patient who ran out of benefits and treatment and killed a foreign president—that shook up the whole healthcare system. Adam had a nightmare about large numbers of the population being found mentally unfit in an evaluation of our country's bridge to the twenty-first century. Maybe it was Sun-Yu's challenge or maybe it was the wine, but they both woke up the next day with a little more humility and awareness.

We, the People

"It is in these more vulnerable populations—the uninsured, Medicaid, and Medicare—that the next big test of managed care will likely occur," continued Sun-Yu the next day. "And it is the people—whether through unions or other coalitions—who are likely to be heard from more and more over the next three years. Until recently, it appears that the values and desires of the people, including the patients, have been neglected in managed care development. We've even seen at times that patients have been told less than previously recommended for informed consent, and that at times clinicians have been influenced not to provide important information about their health plan of choice. Look, John Channing, our consumer representative, and Freddy Famelletti, from the Alliance for the Mentally Ill, have just arrived, so let's hear from them."

"Thanks for involving us again," John commented. "I'm sure you know that different polls found that the number one issue Americans are dissatisfied with—and wanted discussed for the 1996 elections— is healthcare."

"Yes," Freddy added, "and it's somewhat of a surprise to me, although maybe all these years of work by the National Alliance for the Mentally Ill is paying off. Another survey showed that the public is supporting equitable treatment of all illnesses, including brain disorders."

"Besides being ethically just, that should also turn out to be fiscally sound," added Adam. "Federal health reform analyses found that providing more equitable behavioral healthcare coverage might cost $6.5 billion more annually, but would ultimately save $8.7 billion annually in general medical and other indirect costs."

"But it seems like we consumers also need to do more ourselves," added John. "As is often said, real healthcare reform begins with all of us taking responsibility for our own bodies."

"And minds," added Freddy.

"Of course, I was including the mind in the body," John replied with loud laughter. "And we're finally starting to organize nationally in the form of the Consumer Managed Care Network, which has a platform for action consisting of six ethical points:

"One: recovery-oriented values and principles should drive the managed care system.

"Two: consumer rights should be protected at all times.

"Three: consumers should be involved in all aspects of the managed care system.

"Four: quality of care should be paramount.

"Five: services should be affordable and accountable to all consumers.

"Six: quality of the managed care system should be continuously assured.

"Would you all agree with these values?"

"Of course, that's shown in our desire to have you, Freddy, and others involved in all of The Ethical Way's processes," replied Evelyn. "And let's keep the medical savings account alternative to managed care that Sun-Yu mentioned in mind, because that gives the most healthcare power to the people, if they were to spend the money wisely."

"We'll work together with you—and recommend our professional organizations work with you—on a state and national level," added Adam.

"Thank you," Freddy replied. "You're trying to do God's work. If we can get biblical compassion and spirituality back into the marketplace, that should help us get a just behavioral healthcare system that will take good care of our most vulnerable instead of just seeing them as pieces of profit."

"Amen," replied all.

THE ETHICAL WAY TO 2000

"So let's toast the year 2000, when we hope The Ethical Way will be a model for managed behavioral healthcare," Adam suggested to Evelyn after their meeting broke up.

"Yes, it looks like we've found the right ethical balance, not only for ourselves, but hopefully for the managed behavioral healthcare field," Evelyn continued. "Though I'm proud of my own healthcare ethical tradition, I know it had many limitations, including neglect of social costs and considerations, poorly monitored treatment, some greed and other temptations, and a second or third tier of care for the poor and chronically mentally ill."

"Likewise, I'll admit that the business ethics of managed behavioral healthcare, while doing a lot of good in terms of cost savings and bringing attention to how to define good and adequate care, has also fallen ethically short in many ways," added Adam. "Some of the profits and salaries seem almost obscene, research and education have by and large been ignored, utilization review can be more blanket denial than valuable second opinion, and traditional healthcare ethical principles do get compromised without proof of lack of harm to patients, among other ethical concerns."

"And I think our latest discussion and recommendations would suggest a broader balance of relevant ethical principles. So if we were devising a simple equation, it might look like this—" She picked up a piece of scratch paper.

MANAGED BEHAVIORAL HEALTHCARE VALUE =
¼ HEALTHCARE ETHICS, ¼ BUSINESS ETHICS,
¼ GOVERNMENTAL ETHICS, AND ¼ WE-THE-PEOPLE'S VALUES.

"That looks good," said Adam. "As do you. It should remind us what to keep in mind to achieve the right overall ethical balance. How about calling our game up to now a tie?"

"Agreed," Evelyn responded with a hint of embarrassment.

"Fine, can we at least hug on it?" asked Adam.

"Not in public," replied Evelyn with a smile. "A handshake for now. That would be The Ethical Way."

—⁓—

COMMENTARIES ON CHAPTER TEN

Dear Adam and Evelyn:

I can't thank you enough for sending me a copy of the chronicle of The Ethical Way. I must admit that the idea of a description of your first year in a narrative seemed a bit weird at first, but your principles and your story are quite seductive. I've been spending a lot of time with employers, government people, and HMOs, so I guess I can comment on your sense of "future challenges" as you've laid them out in Chapter Ten.

I should also mention that your ideas about future challenges worry me and I think they should worry you too. You formed The Ethical Way in an area that you both know well—personally and professionally. For the most part you've avoided the pitfalls of the utopians but there is still a possibility that you'll find yourselves in the brave new world. You've done a good job in balancing business and health ethics in a specific area of healthcare and you are connected to the real world.

I agree with you that attention to outcomes and research are important, but I expected that you would understand the importance of ongoing, clinically relevant performance measures as a way to decrease variation in practice and to provide real-time feedback to busy clinicians about cost, quality, satisfaction, and effectiveness. After all, "the unexamined practice is not worth doing" (to paraphrase some forgotten psychoanalyst). To hope for knowledge of outcomes sometime in the future may be to deny and displace accountability for today's results.

The anecdotes that you cite—dying babies, suicides, gagged physicians, and so on—are not part of the same reasoned, thoughtful message that you've developed in The Ethical Way. Perhaps you are so involved in your own world, that you have forgotten to test the validity of the conclusions that grow from such stories and to recognize that while these anecdotes make good newspaper stories, they need careful workup before they are accepted as the bottom line.

There is a lot to say about your national perspective and three-year plan. First, I think you should recognize that you have no unique standing. There is no consensus about your life, liberty, and happiness goals, for example. We all know that the Declaration originally read "Life, Liberty, and Property" and the marketplace tells us that property is still important. Further, you go on to elaborate a large role for the federal government on the heels of public rejection of just this sort of centralized control.

To suggest, for example, an oversight role for the Feds before you've explored the questions (oversight of what? by whom? at what cost? with what mission?) seems naive to me. Politicization of the health-care budget means government will increasingly specify medical practice. Medical directors have enough trouble with this. Your allusion to antitrust rules is a good example of your disconnection from the real world: there are excellent, permissive antitrust guidelines now. Asking for a loosening of those guidelines could be asking for permission for professionally led organizations to take undue risks and to put their patients at undue risk.

If you seriously believe that states will slow down the movement of Medicaid patients to managed care, I think you are underestimating the importance of the present political environment and idly dismissing the viewpoints of a large number of the voting public. To do so by pandering to concerns about for-profit managed care companies and the compensation of their CEOs seems unreasoned.

I wish that there were world enough and time to discuss all of this with you. The Ethical Way is a terrific narrative and has a compelling message to deliver. It has an implicit (and at times explicit) message as well: that thought, discussion, careful reading, and collaborative planning can solve serious problems. When it comes to the future and to life outside your Eden, you've drifted away from this message to stake out positions and draw lines. I hope that you'll consider that collaborative problem solving means broad understanding and mutual commitment to change. I think that kind of approach holds promise.

Sincerely,

JOHN M. LUDDEN, M.D.
Senior Vice President of Medical Affairs
Harvard Pilgrim Health Care

———

In my opinion, the author did a reasonable job of posing many of the ethical challenges facing clinicians and administrators under the existing system of mental healthcare, but he missed an excellent opportunity to design a company with a transformed culture of care that incorporated not only the values but the participation of consumers and survivors in the policies, quality improvement, and delivery of services. It is good that the platform of the Consumer Managed Care Network was mentioned in the last chapter, but it seems like an afterthought.

Ultimately, the most cost-effective form of managed care is that which is directed by the consumers themselves, rather than by either the professionals or the MCO. At the National Empowerment Center we call this third generation of managed care *self-managed care*. Under this model the goal of managed care companies is to provide the skills and the environment that promote the capacity of all consumers to control their own treatment and life. This involves opening a number of avenues for consumer involvement in treatment planning such as informed choice, advanced directives, coping strategies, and peer-oriented group therapy. This also involves hiring people who have recovered from mental illness as providers, advisory board members, and trainers. It involves quality improvement through the efforts of consumer and family-run quality evaluation and satisfaction teams.

The most fundamental value of the self-managed care model is a shift in perception such that mental health consumers are seen as capable of recovering through active involvement in their own treatment rather than seen as permanently defective and dependent on perpetual care. To open the eyes of the general public as well as those of clinicians to this hopeful dimension in working with people with mental illness has been the major mission of many hundreds of us who have shown significant recovery. I would recommend that managed care companies of the future draw on these stories of hope.

Another important development in the consumer-survivor movement is the use of holistic and integrative medicine. Underlying this move is an understanding that recovery requires a healing of the deadly split of mind from body that restricts the effectiveness of Western medicine. To design self-managed care strategies, it has been necessary to understand that every mental event is accompanied by a biological event and vice versa. This conceptual step must take place to solve the problem of how to integrate behavioral healthcare with medical healthcare. After all, doesn't all healthcare contain a behavioral dimension? We need to go beyond the unidimensional, either-or thinking of our present medical system. In addition to allowing each consumer to design a more comprehensive healthcare plan, holistic approaches lend themselves to a host of self-care strategies such as exercise, nutrition, and meditation, which are good complements to doctor-directed treatments such as medication and surgery.

Finally, consumer-survivors have found that recovery, like raising a child, requires connection to a caring village. The combination of poor social skills, trauma, lack of resources, and stigma have isolated people with mental health disorders to a frightening degree. The essential element of human warmth is repeatedly cited as necessary for recovery. Consumer-run social clubs and warmlines (a person to call before distress reaches a crisis) often succeed where professionally run facilities have failed because of the importance to recovery of being accepted by a group of peers. The issue of wider community acceptance of people with mental illness should be addressed by everyone in the field.

So an innovative managed care company of the future would, in my view, start with the fundamental principles of recovery gleaned by consumer-survivors, such as hope, self-determination, mind-body integration, and community. Clinical and business practices would then be designed to promote those principles.

The following is a list of articles and videos that are in line with the values of the consumer-survivor movement and promote ethical and cost-effective treatment of mental illness. They may be obtained through the National Empowerment Center, by phoning 1–800–POWER2U or writing 20 Ballard Road, Lawrence MA 01843.

Chamberlin, J. (1979). *On our own: Patient controlled alternatives to the mental health system.* England: Mind Books.

Deegan, P. "Recovery is a journey of the heart." (1995). A sixty-minute video describing Dr. Deegan's recovery from mental illness. Lawrence, MA: National Empowerment Center.

Deegan, P. "Experiential workshop on hearing voices." (1995). A curriculum or a facilitated workshop designed by Dr. Patricia Deegan. Lawrence, MA: National Empowerment Center.

Fisher, D. B. (1995). "Self-managed care: 16 ways that MCO's and their partners can optimally engage consumer/survivors in their recovery." A forty-five-minute video. Lawrence, MA: National Empowerment Center.

Fisher, D. B. (1996). *Self-managed care: You too can heal your "mental illness."* A self-help manual in which Dr. Fisher shares the most important factors in his recovery from mental illness. Lawrence, MA: National Empowerment Center.

Fisher, D. B. "Recovery is for everyone." (1995). A forty-five-minute video. Lawrence, MA: National Empowerment Center.

Zinman, S., Harp, H., and Budd, S. (1987). *Reaching across: Mental health helping each other* (Vol. 1).

Zinman, S., Harp, H., and Budd, S. (1994). *Reaching across: Mental health helping each other* (Vol. 2).

DANIEL B. FISHER, M.D., Ph.D.
Executive Director
National Empowerment Center

—◠◠◠—

> If you want the present and the future to be different from the past, Spinoza tells us, study the past, find out the causes that made it what it was and bring different causes to bear.
>
> —Will and Ariel Durant

One of the greatest ethical challenges to our society in general, and to healthcare in particular, resides in health resource consumption of the aging baby boom generation of Americans born between 1946 and 1964. The arrival of the baby boomers at retirement age in the early twenty-first century will create a tsunami of healthcare demand, making landfall in an environment characterized both by diminishing resources and diminishing political will to satisfy such demands. Universally recognized as an issue of enormous consequence for our society, there has been to date remarkably little productive debate regarding the range of rather stark options, decisions, and policies involved in preparing for this approaching deluge of demand. Issues of a complexity not yet evident in today's ethically challenged healthcare environment are within sight on the horizon.

The crucial issue of rationing of resources and the intensifying debate over whether or not access to healthcare is an entitlement or merely a legal contract covering "lives" (with benefits, exclusions, and limitations) may result in Malthusian, multitiered levels of care with large segments of the population living without coverage. The drive toward resource rationing and restructuring will intensify the ethical questions currently being explored by the author of this work. Others, including Applebaum, Backlar, and their associates, are pursuing the extraordinary potential for conflicts of interest within and among hybrid payer-provider systems, the use of living wills or advanced directives regarding an individual's choice of treatment in the event of mental or physical incapacities, and the distortion of traditional social justice principles when cost is perceived as the sole denominator of the public interest.

The unidimensional focus on cost to the exclusion of other values may also lead to the eroding of traditional behavioral health law, which currently safeguards individual rights, confidentiality, and social justice. As integrated, risk-bearing organized systems begin to move away from supply-side management strategies, demand management approaches will raise new ethical issues over confidentiality and individual human rights to not "live in a reasonably healthy manner" while persisting in "diseases of choice," such as obesity and legal or illegal substance abuse. Should such individuals be involuntarily treated or denied care related to those disorders? Apart from issues of confidentiality, the use of advanced biomonitoring and genetic testing for prevention, early intervention, and maintenance regimes will raise particularly difficult and disturbing ethical questions.

It is clear that future ethical challenges and choices must be informed by an elaborate, advanced multi-axial calculus. Such an ethical quadratic will not inform the ethical deliberations between society, payer, provider, and consumer unless there is a common methodology to define and measure value exchanges between all stakeholders. The ethics of resource allocation, distribution, and the valuation of the impact and return to society, provider, and consumer dictate the necessity of such measures for informed decision making. Current efforts under way to establish common methodologies to assist in ethical, policy, and clinical decision making must be accelerated. Although politically and economically daunting, the basis for ethical deliberation focusing on the distribution of resources requires that cost-effective studies include all societal costs, not just costs for one affected group. General health characteristics of different racial, age, or economic groups must also figure into any calculation of value.

Continued attention must be given to the social compact between business and society in the postcapitalistic age. What duty is owed, to whom, and under what circumstances? What obligation is owed by healthcare providers for noninsured or noncovered individuals in a community? As federal, state, and local governments become the major payers for the majority of the population in the twenty-first century, what will be the balance between return on investment and return on resources raised through public means? To what extent will healthcare be viewed exclusively as a deregulated free market? Will healthcare be viewed if not as an entitlement at least as a public utility, vital to the public safety and health of communities? Healthcare providers, purchasers, and consumers are well advised to inject such ethical concerns and issues into a public policy environment almost entirely dominated by cost and not value parameters.

CHARLES G. RAY
CEO
National Community Mental Healthcare Council

~~~ Chapter Notes

Chapter One

P. 4: national survey of academic chairs of departments of psychiatry on managed care: Moffic, H., Krieg, K., & Prosen, H. (1993). Managed care and academic psychiatry: A national survey. *Journal of Mental Health Administration, 20,* 172–177.

P. 10: Hippocratic Oath: Moffic, H., Coverdale, J., & Bayer, T. (1990). The Hippocratic Oath and clinical ethics. *Journal of Clinical Ethics, 1,* 287–289.

P. 12: several stages of managed care described by Jeremy Lazarus, M.D., in: Wagner, J., & Gartner, C. (1996). Issues in managed care: Highlights of the 1995 Institute on Psychiatric Services. *Psychiatric Services, 47,* 15–20.

P. 12: recent psychiatric conference: Wagner, J., & Gartner, C. (1996). Issues in managed care: Highlights of the 1995 Institute on Psychiatric Services. *Psychiatric Services, 47,* 15–20.

P. 12: help psychiatrists adapt to managed care: Nadelson, C., & Rieder, R. (1995, December 2). Psychiatrists' work in the 21st century. *Psychiatric News,* pp. 3, 14.

P. 15: how a managed care system might develop and struggle with real-life issues: Cohen, J. (1996, March). An awesome responsibility for medical educators. *Academic Physician and Scientist,* p. 8.

Chapter Two

P. 20: Code of Hammurabi: Darr, K. (1987). *Ethics in health services management.* New York: Praeger.

P. 22: James Sabin on how to manage the tensions between the interests of the individual patient and society: Sabin, J. (1994). Caring about patients and caring about money: The American Psychiatric Association Code of Ethics meets managed care. *Behavioral Sciences and the Law, 12,* 317–330. The quoted passage is on p. 317.

P. 22: core principles: The American Psychiatric Association's Council on Psychiatry and Law. (1995, December 2). Ethical practice under managed care. *The Mental Health Canary: The Voice of Psychotherapy.*

P. 23: Eugenio Chavez-Rice's general set of ethical principles in mental health: Chavez-Rice, E. (1982). Appendix: Code of ethical principles in mental health. In H. Moffic & G. Adams (Eds.), *A clinician's manual of mental health care: A multidisciplinary approach.* Menlo Park, CA: Addison-Wesley.

P. 25: the purpose of business: Sherwin, J. (1983). The ethical roots of the business system. *Harvard Business Review, 83,* 183–192.

P. 25: gap between theoretical ethics and business practice: Nash, L. (1981). Ethics without the sermon. *Harvard Business Review, 81,* 78–90.

P. 25: Ethics Check questions: Blanchard, K., & Peale, N. (1988). *The power of ethical management.* New York: Morrow.

P. 25: how a business school should behave toward other organizations, customers, and the environment: Walton, C. (1988). *The moral manager.* Cambridge, MA: Ballinger.

P. 25: business not simply as an acquisitive trade: Zakaria, F. (1987, October 19). Ethics for greedheads. *New Republic,* pp. 18–20.

Chapter Three

P. 35: role of leaders in meeting the challenge of providing compassionate and cost-effective healthcare: Kohles, M., Baker, G., & Donaho, B. (1995). *Transformational leadership: Renewing fundamental values and achieving new relationships in health care.* Chicago: American Hospital Association.

P. 35: how to further imbue the organization with high ethical standards: Reiser, S. (1994, November-December). The ethical life of health care organizations. *Hastings Center Report,* pp. 28–35.

P. 38: ethical and legal problems in Rhode Island: Saeman, H. (1995). Managed care giant faces ouster in Rhode Island. *The National Psychologist, 4* (4), 1–2.

P. 39: related example: Houghton, W. (1994, September). The day I got my walking papers from UBS. *The Mental Health Canary,* p. 2.

P. 39: published response: German, M. (1994, November). United Behavioral Systems: The messenger pigeon and the airline. *The Mental Health Canary,* p. 2.

P. 39: how that process was used to provide a potentially better system: Adams, H. (1993). Harvard Community Health Plan's Mental Health Redesign Project: A managerial and clinical partnership. *Psychiatric Quarterly, 64,* 13–31.

P. 41: other models: Reidy, W. (1993). Staff model HMO's and managed mental health care. *Psychiatric Quarterly, 64,* 33–44.

P. 43: Values Quiz: Walton, C. (1988). *The moral manager.* Cambridge, MA: Ballinger.

Chapter Four

P. 55: undiagnosed mental health disorder: Cummings, N., & Sayama, M. (1995). *Focused psychotherapy.* New York: Brunner/Mazel.

P. 55: fifty years later, it looks like not much has changed, is substantiated in: Fifer, S., et al. (1994). Untreated anxiety among adult primary care patients in a health maintenance organization. *Archives of General Psychiatry, 51,* 740–750. See also: Kaplan, A. (1996). Multicenter-HMO study under way on depression in primary care. *Psychiatric Times, 13* (1), 1, 8–9.

P. 57: numbers answered by high school graduates: Goleman, D. (1996, January 24). Critics say managed-care controls are eroding mental health. *New York Times Health,* p. B7.

P. 58: no available research to answer which mental health discipline is likely to do the most cost-effective triage: Povar, G., & Moreno, J. (1988, September). Hippocrates and the health maintenance organization: A discussion of ethical issues. *Annals of Internal Medicine,* pp. 419–424.

P. 61: mental health checkup: Moffic, H., & Chavez-Rice, E. (1982). Primary preventive methods and the mental health checkup, in Moffic, H., & Adams, G. (Eds.) *A clinician's manual on mental health care: A multidisciplinary approach.* Menlo Park, CA: Addison-Wesley.

P. 64: an approach to medical necessity: Glazer, W. (1992). Psychiatry and medical necessity. *Psychiatric Annals, 22,* 362–366.

P. 65: scholarly discussion of medical necessity: Sabin, J., & Daniels, N. (1994, November-December). Determining "medical necessity" in mental health practice. *Hastings Center Report,* pp. 5–13.

Chapter Five

P. 72: *Time* magazine: Larson, E. (1996, January 22). The soul of an HMO. *Time,* pp. 44–52.

P. 77: informed consent is not a traditional healthcare ethical guideline: Veatch, J. (1995, March-April). Abandoning informed consent. *Hastings Center Report,* pp. 5–12.

P. 81: certain patterns seem to be emerging: Fields, H. (1995). Managed mental health care: Changing the future of mental health treatment. *Journal of Health and Hospital Law, 28,* 344–363.

P. 82: extension of the gag clause: Editorial. (1996, March). Hazardous duty. *The Mental Health Canary,* p. 1.

Chapter Six

P. 93: confidentiality has been a major healthcare guideline since at least the Hippocratic Oath: Moffic, H., Coverdale, J., & Bayer, T. (1990). The Hippocratic Oath and clinical ethics. *Journal of Clinical Ethics, 1,* 287–289. The oath itself is quoted in full on p. 288.

P. 93: most authorities emphasize that confidentiality may be even more crucial in behavioral healthcare: Gutheil, T. (1990). Ethical issues in confidentiality. *Psychiatric Annals, 20,* 605–611. See also: Goldstein, R. (1992). Psychiatric poetic license? Post-mortem disclosure of confidential information in the Anne Sexton case. *Psychiatric Annals, 22,* 341–348.

P. 95: the same psychotherapists who advocated for absolute confidentiality would often comply and write letters on their patients' behalf: Plaut, E. (1974). A perspective on confidentiality. *American Journal of Psychiatry, 131,* 1021–1024.

P. 96: that Sexton case: Middlebrook, D. W. (1991). *Ann Sexton.* Boston, MA: Houghton Mifflin.

P. 96: a Canadian Study in 1980 found numerous releases of confidential personal information to third parties which were not authorized by patients: Hoffman, B. (1981). Confidentiality and health care: The issues. *Canadian Journal of Psychiatry, 26,* 574–576.

P. 96: found that well over half admitted that they had inadvertently breached a patient's confidentiality: Pope, K., Tabachnick, B., & Keith-Spiegel, P. (1987). Ethics of practice. *American Psychologist, 42,* 993–1005.

P. 97: managed care companies ask for more information than third parties traditionally requested: Edwards, H. (1995, November, December). Managed care and confidentiality. *Behavioral Health Management,* pp. 25–27.

P. 99: electronic records can enhance quality of care in several ways: Tracy, N., & Kesser-Hoffman, C. (1996, February). Computerization with increased patient protection. *Behavioral Healthcare Tomorrow,* pp. 28, 40–41.

P. 102: develop a comprehensive organization policy and procedure for appropriate handling of behavioral healthcare information: Wald, J. (1996, February). Best strategies for clinical delivery systems. *Behavioral Healthcare Tomorrow,* pp. 39, 42, 44.

P. 102: access to sensitive medical information: Waller, A., & Darrah, J. (1996, February). Legal requirements for computer security: Electronic medical records and data interchange. *Behavioral Healthcare Tomorrow,* pp. 45–47.

P. 102: sign confidentiality statements: Barrows, R., & Clayton, P. (1996, February). Confidentiality of healthcare records. *Behavioral Healthcare Tomorrow,* pp. 38, 41, 43–44.

Chapter Seven

P. 114: questionable quality: Sturm, R., & Wells, K. (1995). How can care for depression become more cost-effective? *Journal of the American Medical Association, 273,* 51–58.

P. 118: brief historical summary: English, J., Kritzler, Z., & Scherl, D. (1984). Historical trends in the financing of psychiatric services. *Psychiatric Annals, 14,* 322–331.

P. 120: rapid development of private, investor-owned psychiatric hospitals in the 1980s: Rafferty, T. (1984). The case for investor-owned hospitals. *Hospital and Community Psychiatry, 35,* 1013–1016.

P. 121: former for-profit hospitals: Crawford, M. (1995, February). The wake-up call. *Hospitals and Health Networks,* pp. 5, 48.

P. 122: escalation of managed care was inevitable: Stanton, D. (1989). Mental health care economics and the future of psychiatric practice. *Psychiatric Annals, 19,* 421–427.

P. 122: look back to our country's Declaration of Independence: Moffic, H. (1996). Life, liberty, happiness, and managed care. *Psychiatric Services, 47,* 223.

P. 123: managed care financial mechanisms seem to save money: Iglehart, J. (1990, January 11). Managed care and mental health. *New England Journal of Medicine,* pp. 131–135.

P. 124: as good treatment outcomes in managed care: Lazarus, A. (1995). Managed care practice and psychiatric deaths: Must we assign blame? *Administration and Policy in Mental Health, 22,* 457–461.

P. 124: the reluctance of psychoanalysts to publicly discuss fees: Greenson, R. (1967). *The technique and practice of psychoanalysis.* New York: International University Press.

P. 124: clear out some dead wood: (1988). Concern with money may undermine psychoanalysis. *Clinical Psychiatry News, 16* (3), 13.

P. 127: social workers had the highest rate of income increases: Social workers therapy income up. (1995). *NASW News, 40* (5), 1, 10.

P. 127: even under clinician-led managed care systems, financial needs seem paramount: Physician-led MCO's acting like insurance companies. (1996, February). *Behavioral Healthcare Tomorrow,* p. 12.

P. 129: student interns often produced better results than experienced clinicians: Lerner, B. (1972). *Psychotherapy in the ghetto.* Baltimore: Johns Hopkins University Press.

P. 129: teaching time is poorly compensated: Shea, S., et al. (1996, January 18). Compensation to a department of medicine and its faculty members for the teaching of medical students and house staff. *The New England Journal of Medicine,* pp. 162–167.

P. 130: academic centers will need to accept managed care more than they have: Residency directors consider GME financing strategies. (1996, March 1). *Psychiatric News,* pp. 4, 24.

P. 132: increasing copayments has been found to decrease demand in a progressive manner: Simon, G. (1996). Impact of visit co-payments on outpatient mental health utilization by members of a health maintenance organization. *American Journal of Psychiatry, 153,* 331–338.

P. 132: missed sessions are billed for: Blackman, W. (1993). Are psychoanalysis practices ethical? *American Journal of Psychotherapy, 47,* 613–620.

Chapter Eight

P. 137: a joint private and public venture could meld the best of both: Va-based managed care company joins with community mental health centers. (1996, March 25). *Mental Health News Alert,* p. 3.

P. 143: psychological testing: Moreland, K. (1996, February). How psychological testing can reinstate its value in an era of cost containment. *Behavioral Healthcare Tomorrow,* pp. 59–61.

P. 143: no treatment is the treatment of choice: Clarkin, J. (1995, November). When is no treatment the treatment of choice? *Journal of Practicing Psychiatry and Behavioral Health,* pp. 241–243.

P. 144: a lack of treatment readiness: Raskin, R., & Novacek, J. (1996, April). Treatment readiness: A missing link in behavioral healthcare outcomes measurements. *Behavioral Healthcare Tomorrow,* pp. 63–65.

P. 146: Freud and fifteen-minute checks: Houghton, W. (1994, June). Would Freud do 15-minute checks? *Psychiatric Times,* pp. 23–24.

P. 147: case management has a different sort of tradition in community mental health than in managed care: Anthony, W. (1996, April). Managed care case management for people with serious mental illness. *Behavioral Healthcare Tomorrow,* pp. 67–69.

P. 150: recent recommendations on how to do a brief medication check: Blackwell, B. (1996). Anatomy of a med check. *Wisconsin Psychiatrist, 36*(3), 12.

P. 151: lack of firm guidelines of what to do with an individual patient: Gorman, J. (1995–96). Limits of research as a guide to clinical practice. *Progress Notes, 6* (4), 41–42.

P. 152: cost-effective data is so far inconclusive: Sclar, D., et al. (1994). Antidepressant pharmacology: Economic outcomes in a health maintenance organization. *Clinical Therapeutics, 16,* 715–730; Einarson, T., et al. (1995). A model to evaluate the cost-effectiveness of oral therapies in the management of patients with major depressive disorders. *Clinical Therapeutics, 17,* 136–153; Sclar, D., et al. (1995). Antidepressant pharmacology: Economic evaluation of Fluoxetine, Paroxetine and Sertraline in a health maintenance organization. *Journal of International Medical Research, 23,* 395–412.

P. 153: ethically mandatory to recommend: Sabin, J. (1994). A credo for ethical managed care in mental health practice. *Hospital and Community Psychiatry, 45,* 859–860.

Chapter Nine

P. 164: recommended articles: Zusman, J. (1990). Utilization review: Theory, practice, and issues. *Hospital and Community Psychiatry, 41,* 531–536. Hoge, S. (1990). Utilization review: A house divided. *Hospital and Community Psychiatry, 41,* 367–368. Blackwell, B. (1996, March). The pendulum swings. *The Mental Health Canary,* pp. 1–2.

P. 166: appeal approval rate of less than 5 percent: Fields, H. (1995). Managed mental health care: Changing the future of mental health treatment. *Journal of Health and Hospital Law, 28,* 344–363.

P. 166: hypocritical for psychiatrists to complain: Schlesinger, M., Dorwart, R., & Epstein, S. (1996). Managed care constraints on psychiatrists' hospital practices: Bargaining power and professional autonomy. *American Journal of Psychiatry, 153,* 156–160.

P. 167: the most similar medical activity to utilization review may be forensic evaluations: Huge, S. (1995, November). Making allocation decisions in
an environment of constrained resources. *Journal of Practicing Psychiatry
and Behavioral Health,* pp. 255–257.

P. 167: two published accounts: Parlour, R. (1986). Reflections of a CHAMPUS-
APA peer review. *Journal of Clinical Psychiatry, 47,* 71–74. Mohl, P. (1996). Confessions of a concurrent reviewer. *Psychiatric Services, 47,* 35–40.

P. 171: ethical and legal reasons that they are concerned about utilization
review: Gabbard, G., et al. (1991). A psychodynamic perspective on the
clinical impact of insurance review. *American Journal of Psychiatry, 148,*
318–322.

P. 171: case: Blackwell, B. (1994). No margin, no mission. *Journal of the
American Medical Association, 271,* 1466.

P. 172: patients are often surprised: Walter, K. (1995, December 9). Give me
therapy—or else. *The New York Times.*

P. 179: some of the recommendations: Green, S. (1989). The process of
reviewing peers. *General Hospital Psychiatry, 11,* 264–267.

P. 181: individual variation would be neglected: Wickizer, T., Lessler, D., &
Travis, K. (1996). Controlling in-patient psychiatric utilization through
managed care. *American Journal of Psychiatry, 153,* 339–345.

Chapter Ten

P. 185: corporate moral development: Starke, L. (1993). The five steps
of corporate moral development. In M. Ray & A. Rinzler (Eds.), *The new
paradigm in business.* New York: Putnam.

P. 188: fraud by hospitals and clinicians: Caper, P. (1995). Commentary on
managed care. *Public Health Reports, 110,* 682–683.

P. 188: paying less for behavioral healthcare: Tucker, M. (1996, March 20).
The future of psychiatry: Organize or perish. *Clinical Psychiatry News,* p. 20.

P. 191: apparent wide variability in the quality of managed care companies:
Francis, A. (1996, January). The pluses and minuses of managed care. *Journal of Practicing Psychiatry and Behavioral Health,* p. 1.

P. 191: report cards have helped to improve treatment in medicine:
Montague, J. (1996, January 5). Report card daze. *Hospitals and Health
Networks,* pp. 33–36.

P. 194: a managed care initiative: Goplerud, E. (1996, April). Managed care in the public sector: The federal role. *Behavioral Healthcare Tomorrow,* pp. 71–73.

P. 200: six ethical values: Consumer Managed Care Network. (1996, April). Platform for action. *Behavioral Healthcare Tomorrow,* p. 36.

P. 201: Medical savings account alternative: Stock, H. (1994, November 4). Medical savings accounts would return control to consumers. *Psychiatric News,* pp. 15, 24.

P. 202: the right ethical balance: Hartwig, A., & Eichelman, B. (1986). The ethics of mental health practice. *Psychiatric Annals, 16,* 547–552.

—ⁿⁿ⁻ For Further Reading

Beauchamp, T., & Childress, J. (1994). *Principles of medical ethics* (4th ed.). New York: Oxford University Press.

An excellent basic text on bioethical principles.

Blanchard, K., & Peale, N. (1988). *The power of ethical management.* New York: Morrow.

A quick-reading book on how to apply sound ethics to the benefit of any business.

Bollas, C., & Sundelson, D. (1995). *The new informants.* Northvale, NJ: Aronson.

If one wants to read a strong criticism of how societal changes, including managed behavioral healthcare, have affected confidentiality, this is the book.

Darr, K. (1987). *Ethics in health services management.* New York: Praeger.

Though not discussing managed care per se, an excellent overview of the application of healthcare ethics to organizations and administrators. Includes an appendix of different ethical codes for healthcare institutions.

Goldman, W., & Feldman, S. (1993). *Managed mental health care.* San Francisco: Jossey-Bass.

This edited volume produces a nice overview of how managed care has affected a wide variety of private and public sector systems.

Gray, B. (1991). *The profit motive and patient care.* Cambridge, MA: Harvard University Press.

A critique of how pervasive the profit motive became for hospitals and physicians by the 1980s, with a beginning analysis of how managed care may offer some necessary corrections.

Haas, L., & Malouf, J. (1995). *Keeping up the good work: A practitioner's guide to mental health ethics* (2nd ed.). Sarasota, FL: Professional Resource Press.

Though devoting only three pages to managed care, this volume offers a comprehensive discussion of many basic ethical concerns in behavioral healthcare. As a bonus, it includes copies of the codes of ethics for the American Association for Marriage and Family Therapy, American Psychiatric Association, American Psychological Association, and National Association of Social Workers.

Melek, S., & Pyenson, B. (1995). *Capitation handbook.* Washington, DC: American Psychiatric Association.
Offers a detailed analysis, with figures, about what goes into a capitation rate for various behavioral healthcare populations.

Ray, M., & Rinzler, A. (Eds.). (1993). *The new paradigm in business.* New York: Putnam.
This edited volume offers numerous convincing examples of companies and their leaders who are trying to instill new values into the business world.

Reiser, S., et al. (1987). *Divided staffs, divided selves.* Cambridge, MA: Cambridge University Press.
Though lacking managed behavioral health cases, the volume offers interesting case examples of ethical challenges in mental health.

Research Group of the Hastings Center Project on Priorities in Mental Health. (1993, September-October). Minds and hearts: Priorities in mental health services. *Hastings Center Report Special Supplement,* entire issue.
This special issue offers a wide-ranging analysis of prioritizing mental health services, including principles of medical necessity, rationing, and accountability.

Schreter, R., Sharfstein, S., & Schreter, C. (1994). *Allies and adversaries: The impact of managed care on mental health services.* Washington, DC: American Psychiatric Press.
By using a point-and-counterpoint style, this edited volume tries to present both the managed care and clinician points of view about various topics, including one section on ethical issues.

Transcript summary. (1991). Ethics in Managed Care Conference, October 26–29, 1991. Washington, DC: American Psychiatric Association.
Though somewhat difficult to read, and geared to psychiatrists, this transcribed volume presents a real-life discussion of the viewpoints of many participants in 1991 on ethical issues.

~~~ About the Author

H. Steven Moffic, M.D., is currently director of the Managed Care Division of the Department of Psychiatry and Behavioral Sciences at the Medical College of Wisconsin. He is also a professor with tenure in that department as well as in the Department of Family and Community Medicine.

He has spent most of his twenty-year career developing and leading cost-effective systems of behavioral healthcare, ranging from community mental health centers to captitated managed care contracts. Along the way, he has also been an active clinician. He and the systems he has managed have received several awards and recognition for quality of care.

Moffic has published numerous articles on mental health ethics, managed behavioral healthcare, community mental health, and cultural psychiatry. A recent article, "Life, Liberty, the Pursuit of Happiness, and Managed Care," has elicited numerous requests for copies in the United States and foreign countries.

━━ Index